THE

AROMATHERAPY KIT

Essential Oils and How to Use Them

THE
AROMATHERAPY
KIT

Essential Oils and How to Use Them

CHARLA DEVEREUX

Consultant BERNIE HEPHRUN

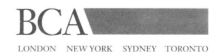

BCA

LONDON   NEW YORK   SYDNEY   TORONTO

Dedication
To the memory of my mother, Selma, who died while
this work was in preparation.

PUBLISHER'S NOTE
The author, publisher and packager cannot accept any responsibility for
misadventure resulting from the use of essential oils, or any other therapeutic
methods that are mentioned in this book.

This edition published 1993
by BCA by arrangement with
HEADLINE BOOK PUBLISHING PLC

CN 6827

10 9 8 7 6 5 4 3 2

AN EDDISON • SADD EDITION
Edited, designed and produced by
Eddison Sadd Editions Limited

Phototypeset in Bembo by Wyvern Typesetting, Bristol, England.
Origination by Columbia Offset, Singapore.
Book printed and bound in Italy by Graphicom Srl.
Oils supplied by Butterbur & Sage Ltd.

CONTENTS

Introduction   6

Chapter 1
Essential Oils   15

Chapter 2
A–Z of Essential Oils   26

Chapter 3
Using Essential Oils   45

Chapter 4
Essential Oils and Beauty Care   68

Chapter 5
Essential Oils and Bodily Health   77

Chapter 6
Essential Oils and the Mind   91

Chapter 7
Your Aromatherapy Kit   96

Glossary   110
Bibliography   110
Useful Addresses   111
Acknowledgements   111
Index   112

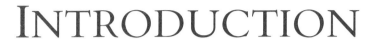

INTRODUCTION

Your *Aromatherapy Kit* consists of a set of five essential oils – Eucalyptus, Geranium, Lavender, Rosemary and Tea Tree – especially selected for their range of properties which can treat a wide variety of conditions, and a manual which tells you how to apply them. Obviously, you will be keen to start using the oils, but before you do it is vital that you read about how to use them safely. The essential oils included in this kit are fully discussed and their uses outlined in chapter seven of this book. Chapters one and three contain all the necessary information for the safe and effective use of the essential oils. This information can also be applied to many other essential oils commonly used in aromatherapy, as discussed in chapter two. Chapters four to six contain a range of charts and information that indicate clearly the essential oils recommended for health, beauty and mental well-being. A glossary is also included. It is suggested that the information in the book be fully understood prior to using the essential oils so that an overall understanding of aromatherapy is obtained. The book can then be used for reference as and when needed.

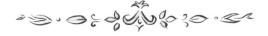

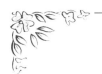

WHAT IS AROMATHERAPY?

The concept that preventative therapy has a vital role to play in the area of complementary medicine is now constantly gaining ground. What this signifies is an attempt to re-establish the connection with our planet that was so naturally enjoyed by our ancestors who had a more synergistic relationship with the earth. Sadly, modern Westernized societies have lost their former awareness of the planet.

Although orthodox medicine has an indisputably important function, the responsibility for maintaining our personal health and well-being is ultimately our own. Our bodies, like all living things, need to be nurtured in order to prosper. As we are integrated into the living processes of earth, it naturally follows that we are dependent on the planet for survival. Our ancestors knew this; they took from and gave back to the earth; but we have severed these connections. Now we must re-establish them to safeguard our future existence.

Preventative medicine is an approach that is available to us all, and plants are among the most precious gifts for this purpose that our planet has to offer. We need to understand, cherish and use them wisely. Aromatherapy, which uses essential oils derived from plant material, is one of the ways we can.

Aromatherapy applies to any use of essential oils that benefits an individual. In order to comprehend the rationale behind aromatherapy, we have to start at the beginning, by understanding the sense of smell itself.

THE SENSE OF SMELL

The olfactory function allows a direct connection to the brain. Sensory cells in the mucous membrane line the nasal cavity and are stimulated by the presence of chemical particles dissolved in the mucus. Fibres of the olfactory nerve run upward from smell receptors in the nasal mucosa high in the roof of the nose, through minute holes in the skull where they enter the olfactory bulb of the brain. The signals are carried to the rhinencephalon (part of the limbic system of the brain concerned with the sense of smell) where the smells are analysed. What is perceived in the brain as an odour is, in fact, the chemical particles. We can register as many as ten thousand different

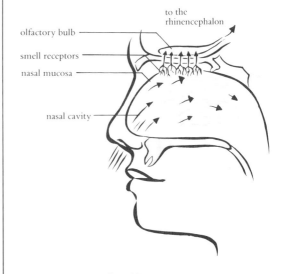

The Olfactory System

fragrances, in contrast to our sense of taste which can register only four types of taste. The sense of smell has by far the greatest capacity. Without it, foods would taste quite bland. This may seem odd, but we need only think of how tasteless food is when a cold has blocked our nasal passages.

Ironically, of our five senses, that of smell is the least developed. This was not always the case: a keen sense of smell was an asset to our ancestors, and was used for hunting game and detecting dangers. This sense is still very important to most creatures; only in modern human beings has it generally become dulled.

Today, we tend to use our sense of smell subconsciously and most of the time we are unaware of the smells around us. What we notice are sudden differences which can often trigger other responses. The smell of smoke or gas, when we are not expecting it, will quickly send us in search of the source. As the limbic system, a centre for emotions, is connected to the hypothalamus, which controls the whole hormonal system through the pituitary gland, it is logical that smells should produce many different responses including anger, comfort, anxiety, sensuality and even fear. The smell of baking bread in the oven is likely to make us feel hungry. Likewise, the smell of rotten eggs can make us feel nauseous. A certain fragrance can awaken a long-forgotten memory as the limbic system is also associated with the establishment of memory patterns. We often link a smell to past events irrespective of the present circumstance in which the smell is manifesting. Frankincense, for example, can have a strong association with church for many people. Patchouli, to a large segment of the population, is a fragrance associated with the 'swinging sixties', and the age of flower power. Smells can evoke positive or negative memories. A certain smell can seem unpleasant, not necessarily because of its fragrance, but because of the memory it evokes. The smell of Lavender or Rose may be comforting because it has an association with the perfume worn by someone special to you.

We can thus begin to see the potential effectiveness of aromatherapy. Indeed, smelling essential oils is considered to be an art. It takes a highly trained individual to be able to distinguish the subtle differences between various qualities of essential oils. In the fragrance business, this person is known as a 'nose'. The 'nose' can fairly quickly determine the quality, origins and indeed the authenticity of an essential oil. It is important to remember though, that not all the components of an oil necessarily have an individual odour. Because of this, the smell on its own cannot fully determine the purity or quality of the oil.

There are two traditional methods of smelling oils: 'organoleptic' and 'sensory analysis'. The organoleptic approach is based solely on the smell and so is achieved by feeling more than analysis. Therefore it is not strictly objective, as the sense of smell will, of course, vary from person to person. It is also difficult to know whether or not the evaluation is coloured by any external factors. In short, this method may be a sound guide, but ultimately it cannot guarantee the quality of an essential oil. For that, more in-depth analysis is required.

In sensory analysis exacting tests are applied, which detect possible contaminates present in an essential oil. The test conditions and environment are controlled to eliminate any variable factors. For example, temperature can have a great effect on the odour of an oil. Basically, the colder the temperature the less smell most oils will produce.

If the quality or purity of an essential oil interests you, then sensory analysis is the most precise method of assessment; however, if you are more concerned about the actual scent, then the organoleptic technique is quite adequate. When smelling essential oils it is best to clear the nose first. This can be done by taking a deep breath and then rapidly exhaling in a series of short spurts. If you are smelling more than one essential oil, remember to clear your nose between sniffs. Because of their strength, it is probably best not to smell more than four oils at one session. Many of them have a tendency to linger in the air and can affect how you perccive the smell of other oils. If you are wearing perfume it can also interfere with your evaluation. Obviously, the fewer external smells present in the environment, the better.

You may want to keep a record of your smell evaluation. This can easily be done by writing down the essential oil name (including the botanical name and origin) and your impression of the smell: what it smells like, how it makes you feel, any memories it stirs up. You may also want to include the supplier's name for future reference. This can be useful in comparing oils from other sources or batches. In this way you can begin to develop your own personal 'nose'.

AROMATHERAPY THROUGH THE AGES

Aromatherapy has a long history. Various parts of plants have been utilized for religious, medicinal and cosmetic purposes by numerous civilizations through the ages. One of the first uses of aromatherapy was probably as a result of the smoke produced by burning plants. This process was among the earliest recorded forms of treatment, and was used mainly to get rid of evil spirits, for it was traditionally thought that disease was caused by an evil spirit inhabiting the sick person's body. The gradual association between the healing of various conditions and the aroma of certain plants might well have served as the foundation for the healing art we today call aromatherapy.

In ancient civilizations, certain plants were considered sacred and used as offerings in ritual practice, often by burning them. Remains of incense have been found in Egypt dating back to about 1500 BC. Incense was considered to be the food of the gods. Plants considered to be sacred were thought to have special powers, and so the connection between holy plants and healing was an obvious one to make. It is still enshrined in the modern

English word 'health', which is cognate with 'holiness' (wholeness). Much of traditional shamanic practice is based on this principle. The shaman was the person in a tribe who knew how to heal and what every herb and plant could be used for. He often used certain powerful plants to achieve the trancelike state necessary to enter the Otherworld in order to obtain healing from the ancestors or the spirits, or to mediate on behalf of tribal members. Tribal peoples had a strong connection with nature and relied on their senses and instinct, something which is very difficult for our sophisticated modern society to understand.

Sometime during the Neolithic or 'new stone age' period (prior to 4000 BC) in the East, as well as in some parts of Europe, the process of extracting fatty oil from various plants by means of pressing seems to have been discovered. This period in prehistory also marks the time when nomadic life was replaced by a more settled existence and tribes began to cultivate land, slowly replacing the need for hunting and gathering. At the same time, the building of sacred monuments was started. In the rituals connected with these, it seems probable that hallucinogenic plants or fungi were ingested. It is chronicled, for instance, that the ancient Scythians threw cannabis onto hot stones and inhaled the vapour with 'howls of pleasure'. The residue of hallucinogenic plants has been found at numerous prehistoric sites. There is some anthropological evidence to suggest that using plants in this manner may have provided an important and particularly powerful way in which early people were able to communicate with other forms of nature as well as with other realms of existence.

Over long periods of time the various properties of herbs would have been discovered. The toxicity levels of plants were slowly understood; some were avoided completely while others were used with caution and care. Chinese medicine, which encompasses a vast knowledge of plant properties, is an important aspect of Chinese civilization, and has been for thousands of years. The Chinese probably have the most comprehensive written record for the medicinal use of herbs.

Unguents or ointments were used in antiquity, particularly in hot dry climates like Egypt where using oils on the body seems to have been an important part of the lifestyle and health practices. Papyri have been discovered dating back to 2551–28 BC recording the medicinal use of herbs. Many vessels have been found that, due to their shape, are believed to have been used to hold oils. Later discoveries of papyri confirm that much was known about the properties of herbs and their applications. Remnants of solidified Frankincense were found in a pot in the tomb of Tutankhamun. Other aromatics known to have been used by the ancient Egyptians include Cedarwood, Coriander, Juniper and Myrrh. These oils were used for many purposes: medicinal, ritualistic as well as cosmetic. For example, Cedarwood was one of the ingredients used in the mummification process. It seems that the best-preserved mummies were those in which large amounts of various oils were used. It followed, then, that these oils would also be used in cosmetics for their rejuvenating properties. There is some evidence which suggests that the Egyptians knew how to extract oil by means of distillation; however, it seems that most of the oils were produced by

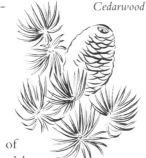

Cedarwood

infusion of the plant in a fatty oil which was then boiled. The perfume would evaporate and become fixed in the fat.

A clay tablet from 1800 BC Babylon proves that trade in oils was going on. Cedarwood, among other oils, was mentioned.

The use of essential oils was one of the many things that the ancient Greeks learned from the Egyptians, particularly the art of perfumery. Wall carvings at the temple of Edfu, Egypt show a substance, possibly oil, being taken from flowers. However, if the Egyptians did know how to distil oil from plants, this information was not passed on to the Greeks.

Many of the perfumes were used for their medicinal properties as well as for cosmetics. The stimulating and sedative properties of a number of plants were recognized.

The recipes for a number of these medicinal perfumes were inscribed on marble tablets in the Greek healing temples of Asklepios and Aphrodite. Asklepios (*Aesculapius*), a son of

Apollo, was a Greek god of healing and there were over 300 Asklepions – centres of healing – dedicated to him, the main one being at Epidaurus in Greece. Vessels for burning incense were found at some of these healing centres. The symbol of Asklepios was a staff with a snake coiled around it, known as the 'caduceus'. In mythology, the snake is associated with the finding of therapeutic herbs. It seems that this curious association dates back to around 2000 BC, when Gilgamesh, a legendary ruler in Mesopotamia, went in search of a herb which he believed would bring eternal life, releasing men from sickness and death. He found the herb at the bottom of the sea. On his way back, Gilgamesh made the fatal mistake of leaving the herb of life on the bank of a lake while he bathed. A snake saw the herb, devoured it and immediately shed its skin, then crawled away. This shedding of the skin was seen as the symbol of rejuvenation, and so the snake came to represent healing. The Hippocratic oath is based on the Asklepian healing tradition, and even today physicians all over the world still ascribe to the principles of the tradition of which the caduceus is still the symbol.

The knowledge obtained by the Greeks was expanded and later used by the Romans. They used preparations from oils on their bodies, clothes, beds and in their homes. It is interesting to note that the word 'perfume' comes from the Latin, *perfumum*, which means 'through smoke'. This would, of course, have originally referred to the use of incense.

The ritual use of oil for anointing someone

indicated that the person had entered a new status or level of initiation. This was a practice widely performed in Judaism. The oil used for anointing kings was supposed to have originally been prepared by Moses. The term 'messiah' comes from the Hebrew word 'mashiach' which means 'anointed'. To anoint, of course, means to rub or massage.

In the tenth century AD, Avicenna (*ibn-Sina*), an Arabian alchemist, discovered the method of distillation. The first essential oil to be extracted was from roses.

Lavender

Rosewater became a popular scent and found its way to Europe during the Crusades. By the end of the twelfth century, perfumes were being manufactured in Europe and by the end of the thirteenth century Lavender had become a popular scent.

The use of plant medicine by physicians was common practice throughout the Middle Ages. In the thirteenth century the use of distillation of plants was encouraged with essence of Rosemary being one of the first to be isolated. Soon afterwards, oils of Lavender and Aspic (Spike Lavender) were also being produced. In 1551, Adam Lonicir wrote a book called *Kräuterbuch* (Herb Book) which stressed the medicinal nature and importance of many herbs and seed oils. By the sixteenth century over seventy essences were being made and used in per-

fumes and cosmetics. However, by the seventeenth century scientists discovered how chemical substances could be used in medicine and it was not long before they were added to and then fully replaced natural essences. One of the reasons for this was that the chemical substances were more powerful and so took less time to effect a cure. Intriguingly, some people may not even realize that plant extracts form the original basis for many of today's 'modern medicines'!

The term 'aromatherapie' comes from R.-M. Gattefossé, a French chemist who worked with essential oils in cosmetics. In 1928, he published a book discussing the use of essential oils in dermatology. In it he stressed the use of 'natural complexes', having found that individual components of a plant were not as effective as the combination which makes up the whole essence. He became interested in the subject as a result of immersing his hand in oil of Lavender after severely burning it in a laboratory explosion. To his surprise his hand healed in a very short time, did not become infected and the burn left no scar. Other French scientists and doctors have continued to study essential oils and only recently have some of these works been translated into English and other languages.

An aromatherapy clinic was set up in Los Angeles in 1938 by M. Godissart, a colleague of Gattefossé, where cures were reportedly taking place for a variety of ailments including skin cancer, gangrene and facial ulcers.

Jean Valnet, a medical practitioner inspired

by Gattefossé's work, came to realize the incredible potential of using herbs when he was treating wounds during World War II. His book, *Aromatherapie*, was published in 1964. Dr Valnet's work was translated into English in 1982 under the title *The Practice of Aromatherapy*. It is due to his work that aromatherapy today is increasingly accepted as a viable complementary therapy.

Marguerite Maury, an Austrian biochemist, is also recognized as an important figure in pioneering the modern approach to aromatherapy. Her style of treatment combined the oriental art of massage with the properties of the essential oils. Her main interest was skin care but she soon realized the overall healing potential of essential oils. She set up the first aromatherapy clinic in London.

Properties from plant essences are currently used in many pharmaceutical preparations. Yet there is still a lingering resistance by orthodox medicine to fully recognize the contribution that essential oils (used in their natural state) have to offer, despite their long tradition. One of the main arguments is that their mode of action is not fully understood. In other words, it cannot be scientifically broken down.

Today a growing number of practitioners and researchers in the orthodox medical establishment are starting to take aromatherapy seriously, at least in concept, if not in name. Dr Susan Schiffman, a professor of medical psychology at Duke University in the United States, has been conducting research on scents and believes that smell can promote relaxation better than visualization techniques. She recognizes that certain stimulating odours do actually affect alertness. She has also been examining the effects of odour on violence.

The scent of Lavender has been used in some hospital wards. In addition to giving a pleasant smell, it helps to prevent infection. In Japan, Peppermint has been used to scent office space as it is said to increase concentration. Fragrance has long been used in certain shops to create a mood and pleasant environment which help to encourage shoppers to stay longer and hopefully to spend more!

The Fragrance Research Fund is a charitable organization based in New York, dedicated to facilitating the study of the sense of smell and the behavioural influence of scent. They supported a study in conjunction with Memorial Sloan-Kettering Cancer Center in New York where it was found that 'Fragrance can be used to reduce the anxiety and distress patients may experience during a widely used medical procedure'. Memorial Sloan-Kettering is the world's largest private institution devoted to advancing the prevention, diagnosis and treatment of cancer.

AROMATHERAPY TODAY

Finally, how can we benefit from aromatherapy today?

There are a growing number of people who are turning to complementary medicine to augment their choice of healing techniques. According to a 1989 survey, cited in the *International Journal of Aromatherapy*, an increasing number of people in Britain, if given the appropriate information and the choice, would like to have complementary therapies incorporated into the National Health Service. A good sign in this direction is the growing number of NHS physicians who are already including homoeopathy and acupuncture in their medical practices.

There are a number of other therapies like aromatherapy that lend themselves equally to use as both preventative and curative medicine. The Indian system of *Ayurveda* is an excellent example of this. It encompasses science, religion and philosophy, providing practical knowledge of self-healing in allowing for basic medical needs to be fulfilled by daily diet. In Chinese medicine the use of herbs for healing is combined with philosophy and nutrition – all three are regarded as equally important.

Massage is another therapy that can be used preventatively. It benefits the body by

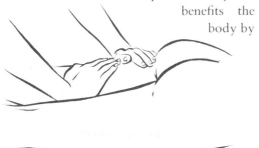

both relaxing the muscles and stimulating blood circulation at the same time. In fact, massage is probably one of the oldest forms of medical treatment. The importance of touch

has been shown to have profound positive effects. Children who receive a lot of physical contact through hugging and other forms of touch tend to be better balanced. They instinctively want to touch and be touched. Touch is both reassuring and comforting. This is true for adults as well, of course! Massage is excellent for relieving tension and soothing anxiety as well as for sore muscles. If just a few minutes of massage around the neck and shoulder area can make a world of difference, imagine what a whole body massage can do! The 'back street massage parlour' connotation that has for too long sullied the modern view of massage is, thankfully, slowly being eroded as the true benefits of massage are being recognized and utilized by mainstream society. The idea, of course, is to alleviate stress and tension before they manifest themselves in other ways which can result in various diseases. Massage is one of the best ways to achieve this.

By combining massage with the use of essential oils almost magical results can be achieved. A regular aromatherapy treatment from a qualified therapist can help keep the body in tip-top condition, by stimulating its own natural healing processes, and freeing it from tension and stress, which is so important for our late twentieth-century lifestyle. This is just one way in which aromatherapy can be employed; in the following pages you will be introduced to numerous other techniques through which you can enjoy the healing benefits of essential oils.

Chapter 1

ESSENTIAL OILS

Essential oils are considered by many to be the hormones or life-force of a plant. They are extracted from a variety of plant parts, such as the flowers, leaves, wood, resin and twigs. The method of extraction depends on the part of the plant from which the oil is being taken; the various methods are discussed later in this chapter. The plants from which essential oils are extracted come from all over the world, and only top quality oils are suitable for aromatherapy purposes. These oils are used by properly trained therapists to help treat a broad spectrum of physical, mental and psychosomatic conditions. Although just smelling them can have the power to alter a person's mood or mental state, they can be used effectively in a number of other ways.

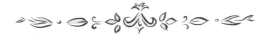

THE NATURE OF ESSENTIAL OILS

Essential oils are extremely concentrated and so should only be used in very small quantities. Although they are called oils, they do not have a greasy texture, and their consistency can range from very watery to syrup-like density. Most essential oils will evaporate totally if left exposed to the air.

An essential oil will not always have the same healing properties as the whole plant from which it comes. This is because there may be a number of active compounds in the original plant that are not present after distillation. Many oils do, however, have antiseptic and anti-bacterial properties and have been shown in laboratory tests to kill bacteria on contact. Chamomile and Lavender, for example, are known to be more powerful as antiseptics than phenol (a man-made disinfectant) when applied to infected wounds.

By using essential oils, and indeed herbs, we are making use of the whole plant as opposed to stripping out one or more of its constituents. For example, menthol is extracted from Peppermint and extensively used in the pharmaceutical industry, along with other mostly synthetic chemical ingredients, to produce cold, flu and digestive aids. Peppermint

Peppermint

itself is a very effective carminative, which helps with digestive disorders as well as being antiseptic when dealing with congestion caused by excessive catarrh. Through the use of the whole plant, be it as a tea or oil, the cause of the problem (blocked sinuses, mental fatigue, etc.) is also worked on. It really makes more sense to use a completely natural remedy than a synthetically created product which is only designed to alleviate the symptoms.

Thyme oil is another example. Both thymol and carvacrol, two of the many constituents of the plant, are isolated and used extensively in the pharmaceutical industry. Another interesting feature of Thyme oil is that it will act as either a stimulant or a relaxant, depending on what is required at the time. This quality is found in a number of other essential oils. Both Geranium and Ylang Ylang, for example, have a balancing action on sebum production and are therefore effective for both dry and oily skin types. *Geranium* (Sebum is an oil produced by the sebaceous glands and provides a thin film over the skin which slows the evaporation of moisture.)

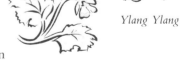

Ylang Ylang

A nineteenth-century French perfumier,

Piesse, devised a system which categorized odours to a scale of top, middle and base notes corresponding to notes on the musical stave. These categories also determine the length of time it takes the fragrance to evaporate. The quickest evaporating oils are called top notes and their scent lasts for minutes 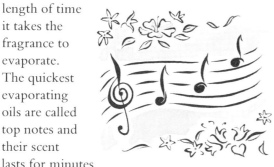 rather than hours. When smelling a blend or perfume, the top note is the first scent you will be aware of. Top note oils tend to be stimulating and energizing. Next come middle note oils whose aroma lasts several hours. These oils give a blend its main characteristics. They have a balancing and harmonizing quality. Oils whose fragrance lasts longest are classified as base notes and they are calming and relaxing in nature. The base notes are the easiest to identify and include Myrrh, Patchouli and Sandalwood. Classification of top notes and middle notes sometimes overlaps and is dependent upon seasonal variations that occur to each new crop.

The molecular structure of essential oils means that they can be easily absorbed through the skin and mucous membranes. Therefore they enter the bloodstream quite rapidly; however, they are also eliminated quickly and so will usually be out of the body between four and six hours after absorption.

Temperature can have an effect on the storage of certain essential oils. If the air is too cool, citrus oils can become cloudy. This is also true for Ylang Ylang. A number of oils will become thicker in cold temperature; Rose Otto in particular will solidify.

Although the basic components will remain the same, the properties of essential oils can differ for a number of reasons. Essential oil taken from two plants of the same species but grown in different parts of the world, or at differing altitudes, will usually show different ratios of the same components. Even plants grown in the same area can change from season to season. These changes occur as a result of variation in soil and climatic conditions, which have an effect on the proportions of the various constituents found in the essential oil. When there is a significant difference which remains constant for a number of seasons in a particular species of plant grown in a particular place, the essential oil from that plant may be classified as a 'chemotype' distinguishing it from the 'standard' oil normally produced by the particular plant species in that area. The effects of seasonal variations on a plant can also have an effect on the aroma of the oil it produces. This does not usually affect the quality of the oil. In fact, the purity of an essential oil may well be more questionable if it has the exact same fragrance from year to year. Synthetically prepared smells are easy to keep constant; it is nature that creates variations.

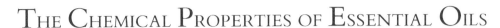

THE CHEMICAL PROPERTIES OF ESSENTIAL OILS

Constituents of essential oils are classified according to chemical or functional groupings. An essential oil may contain more than one hundred components. (The main constituents of each essential oil discussed in this book are indicated by group, in chapter two as part of the information provided in the A–Z listing.) The various chemical groups included are given below with a brief description of their function.

ACIDS

Acids are known to speed up chemical reactions and usually have antiseptic and diuretic properties. They can help to lower fevers.

ALCOHOLS

Solvent action (a liquid which is able to dissolve a substance to form a solution) is the main characteristic of this group. They tend to provide an energizing effect as well as having anti-viral, antiseptic and anti-bacterial properties. Essential oils with a high proportion of alcohols are considered to have a low toxicity level and are relatively safe for general use. These oils include Lavender, Geranium, Tea Tree, Neroli and Rosewood.

ALDEHYDES

These are used in the preparation of solvents, and are often responsible for the scent of a plant. They seem to be the main constituents of Lemon, Lemongrass and Melissa.

ESTERS

These components are formed by condensation of an acid with an alcohol. They are used in flavourings and perfumes as they tend to have a rather fruity fragrance. They usually have sedative and anti-spasmodic properties. There are many esters and when they are found in an essential oil it is usually in small amounts. Oils containing esters include Clary Sage and Lavender.

KETONES

Ketones resemble aldehydes, but are less reactive, providing a solvent action. They help determine the main characteristics of the essential oil in which they occur. Ketones assist in balancing the flow of mucus. It is generally felt by most aromatherapists that oils containing a fair amount of ketones such as Hyssop and Sage, can be hazardous and should be used with care. It is for this reason we suggest that these oils, discussed in the A–Z section, should only be used under the guidance of a qualified aromatherapist. Some oils contain the ketone cineole which can, depending upon the concentration, cause significant burning to mucous membranes if accidentally ingested. These oils include Ginger, Peppermint and Rosemary.

PHENOLS

These are weak acids which have disinfectant and anti-bacterial as well as stimulating properties. They help to cleanse wounds and treat inflammations. They are also useful as pain-killers. Thyme is an example of an essential oil with these attributes. Oils containing these chemicals can be irritating, so they should only be used in low dosages. We recommend throughout this book that they only be used under the guidance of a qualified aromatherapist.

SESQUITERPENES

A number of properties have been attributed to this group of chemicals including anti-inflammatory, anti-spasmodic and stimulating to the immune system. It is azulene, a sesquiterpene, that gives Chamomile, particularly German Chamomile, its distinctive blue colour. Other sesquiterpenes are commonly found in many of the flower oils.

TERPENES

Terpenes are present in most essential oils; they are unsaturated hydrocarbons which are partly responsible for the scent that a plant produces, and can vary from season to season depending on the concentration.

METHODS USED TO EXTRACT ESSENTIAL OILS

There are a number of methods used to extract essential oils from the plant material in which they originate.

STEAM DISTILLATION

This method is the most common form of extraction. The plant parts to be used are usually placed on a grid, and steam at about 110°C is fed in. The essence is released from the plants in the form of a vapour which is then directed through a pipe, along with the steam, passing through cooling tanks which cause the vapour to become liquid. The steam condenses into water. The essence from the vapour (the essential oil) normally floats on this watery distillate, as it is lighter in weight, allowing it to be separated out easily. There are a few

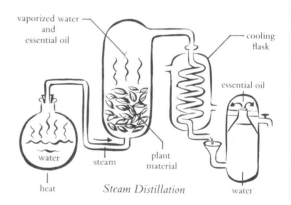

Steam Distillation

essential oils, however, that are heavier than water, Vetivert is an example. For faster results, hydrodiffusion, the application of gentle pressure – usually a vacuum – is used during steam distillation.

ENFLEURAGE

Enfleurage was the traditional and preferred technique for extracting the finest quality essential oil from Jasmine. This is because the delicate flower cannot withstand the heat used in the distillation method due to its detrimental effect on their fragrance. In this method the flower petals are sprinkled over purified fat which absorbs the essence. When the petals fade they are removed and new ones sprinkled over in their place. This process can go on for a number of weeks until the fat reaches its saturation level. The fat, after all of the petals have been removed, is diluted in alcohol and vigorously vibrated for about 24 hours, to separate out the essential oil. These essential oils are known as pomades.

EXPRESSION

This technique is used to extract the essential oils from the outer rind of fruit by pressure. The pulp and white pith are removed, either by scooping them out or by peeling the rind away. In either case the best quality is still obtained by hand. The rind is then squeezed and the liquid from it is left to stand for a while to allow the oil to rise to the surface so that it can be easily removed.

EXTRACTION

The most concentrated of essences is produced by extraction. The flowers are placed on perforated metal trays which are in turn placed in hermetically sealed containers. At one end is a solvent tank, at the other is a vacuum still. A liquid solvent slowly flows over the flowers, dissolving the essential oil as it drains into the still. The solvent, which is recycled after it is distilled, leaves a semi-solid substance (called 'concrete') which contains the aromatic material and natural plant waxes from the flowers. The wax is removed by vibrating the substance in alcohol. What remains is a high quality 'absolute'.

MACERATION

This method can be used at home as long as you have a good supply of suitable herbs or flowers. To prepare essential oil using this technique, the leaves or petals of a plant are placed in a clean jar, filling it about one-third of the way. The rest of the jar is filled with a quality carrier oil (Almond or Grapeseed are good choices). The mixture must be tightly covered to prevent it turning rancid due to oxidation, and it must be kept in a warm, dark place allowing enough time for various properties from the plant

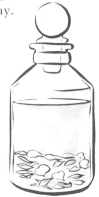

Maceration

material, including the fragrance, to be absorbed into the oil. When the plant material turns brown, it should be replaced with fresh foliage. This can be done several times depending on the concentration you require. After the mixture is strained it will be ready for use. If kept tightly sealed and stored in a dark place it can last for several months.

PERCOLATION

Percolation is a new method as yet not widely in use. It is similar to distillation, except that the steam is produced above the plant material and percolates down through it. The steam and vapours then run, via a pipe, through a series of tanks, each one cooler than the last causing condensation. The remainder of the process is similar to the distillation method. The advantage of percolation over distillation seems to be the ability to extract oil from tough material, such as woods, because it reduces the processing time. Flower waters such as Rose, Neroli and Lavender are by-products of the distillation process.

CAUTION IN THE USE OF ESSENTIAL OILS

Essential oils are by nature very concentrated and so, like any strong substance, they can cause problems if used carelessly.

It is important not to use more than the recommended dosages of essential oils. If you are unsure about the dosage, it is always best to consult a qualified aromatherapist before using the oil. Some oils, when used in excess, can actually cause contra-indications rather than producing the desired effect. This occurs particularly when using essential oils derived from herbs. For instance, Basil is stimulating for the mind, but when too much is used it can have a stupefying effect. Again, although Black Pepper can stimulate urination, when taken in excess it can be damaging to the kidneys. Similarly, Juniper Berry, another essential oil known for its diuretic property, can cause urine retention if taken in excess. Like so many things in life, a little of something can be helpful while too much can have the opposite effect. To paraphrase Paracelsus, the Swiss physician, 'The poison is the dose'. This is, of course, the under-lying principle in homoeopathy, which utilizes microdoses of substances, often from plants, to stimulate the immune system. Each remedy is specially prepared to suit the in-

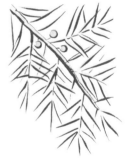

Juniper

dividual needs of the recipient. The system is based on the theory that 'like cures like'. This means that the remedies are actually capable of producing symptoms of the particular disease being treated. So, the homoeopathic therapist endeavours to find a substance that would cause in overdose similar symptoms to those the patient is experiencing. This substance is then given as the remedy, although in very minute amounts. It is interesting to note that this 'law of similars' is also a basic principle of physics. The way to recharge a weak magnet is

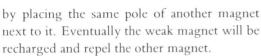

by placing the same pole of another magnet next to it. Eventually the weak magnet will be recharged and repel the other magnet.

Use of essential oils for treatment of specific complaints is best done under the guidance of a certified aromatherapist. For example, there are a range of oils including Lavender, Marjoram and Chamomile, that are beneficial for menstrual pain which can be effectively used in a hot compress or massage blend. However, as their individual actions are quite specific, care needs to be taken when choosing. Clary Sage, for example, is also effective for relieving menstrual pains; however, it is also an emmenagogue so should not be used if menstrual flow is normal or heavy. There are a number of other oils that fall into this category (see chapter five).

Unfortunately, a situation or condition can actually worsen before it begins to improve when starting an aromatherapy treatment. This is, alas, a common occurrence in various forms of natural healing. Juniper, for example,

is very effective for acne; however, it can initially make the symptoms worse. Juniper stimulates the elimination of toxins, so as the toxins are being 'awakened' they can cause disturbance to an already scarred skin. Only when the toxins have been expelled will the skin's condition start to improve.

Essential oils should never be taken internally except under the guidance of a qualified aromatherapist. Some oils are toxic, and although relatively high dosages would have to be ingested in most cases for serious effects to occur, it is wise to err on the side of caution. It is imperative that bottles of essential oil are kept out of the reach of children for this reason. Also as a basic precaution, all essential oil bottles should be fitted with a flow-restrictor to help avoid excess amounts of oil being dispensed accidentally.

Some essential oils should not be used when taking homoeopathic remedies as they can reduce the effectiveness. It is always best to consult a qualified practitioner.

HEALING PROPERTIES OF ESSENTIAL OILS

Each plant contains an abundance of constituents. Many, but not all, are known. The healing properties of the plant depend to a large extent on all of the constituents working together. In modern medicine a constituent that is known to have a particular healing property is often isolated from the plant and processed, usually along with a number of synthetic ingredients, to form a manufactured

drug. Very often the man-made drug has a number of side-effects that, in some cases, can be worse than the original ailment. Although natural curatives usually take longer to work, they are gentler on the body and often more effective than the processed remedy. It is truly a case of the whole being of greater value than the actions of any of the individual parts. Furthermore, it does not always follow that if a particular constituent known to be a sensitizing agent is present in an essential oil then the oil itself is sensitizing. In many cases the combination of a sensitizing agent with other constituents cancels out the sensitizing effect. Nature is definitely the world's superior chemist and pharmacist!

In *The Practice of Aromatherapy*, Dr Jean Valnet talks about the value of using essential oils in their natural state as opposed to using only the main constituents of a particular plant. Lemon essential oil, for example, he believes is 'second to none' as far as its antiseptic and anti-bacterial properties are concerned. Studies have shown that the vapours from natural Lemon essential oil, for example, can neutralize a number of infectious bacteria in a very short period of time. Valnet states that 'The *whole* natural essence is found to be more active than its principle constituent. Moreover, those constituents which form a smaller percentage of the whole are found to be more active than the principal constituent.' This, as he indicates, is an example of synergy (a number of things working in co-ordination with one another). Valnet suggests that Lemon essential oil is useful for a variety of illnesses, but it must be remembered that he is speaking as a professional medical doctor; an aromatherapist is not able to make such claims. It can only be hoped that more people in the medical profession will take an interest

Lemon

in his work and set about furthering it.

An individual essential oil can have a variety of uses based on the number of constituents it contains. Equally there is usually a wide choice of essential oils that can be used for a particular condition. This allows for other factors, like personal preference, to be considered when choosing which essential oils to use.

Some oils contain properties that are harmonious to our own body chemistry. Fennel, for example, has been known through the

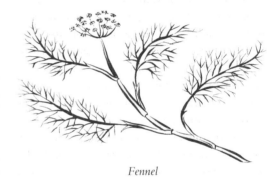

Fennel

ages for its positive effects on the female reproductive system. Modern research indicates that this is due to a hormone in the plant which has a similar action to oestrogen. During menopause, there is a reduction in the level of oestrogen production which can cause a number of symptoms to occur including dizziness, headaches, anxiety, sweats and insomnia. Fennel can be useful during menopause to help moderate the fluctuation in oestrogen levels.

Consult chapter two for further information on the conditions that each oil treats.

ASSESSING THE PURITY OF ESSENTIAL OILS

It is important to be sure that the essential oils you use for aromatherapy purposes are naturally derived and have been produced by a single distillation or extraction process with nothing added or manipulated. Although a product may be marked 'essential oil', that does not necessarily mean it is pure! Some companies, in order to save money, adulterate certain essential oils with a cheaper oil. Rose, for example, can be diluted with Geranium or Palmarosa (both less expensive essential oils). These can still be called natural aromatherapy products, but the price often reveals the truth. If Rose and Jasmine are close in price to Lavender or Geranium, for example, you can safely guess they are not of the quality necessary for aromatherapy purposes.

Synthetic oils are available, often known as Nature Identicals, which actually resemble the natural oil both in major components as well as aroma. The key here, of course, is the word 'major' as it is impossible to duplicate *all* the components.

It is possible for detailed analytical information to be obtained from a small sample of an essential oil by means of chromatography. This technique checks the 'fingerprint' of the oil in question by separating out the various substances and comparing them to the known components of the essential oil as it occurs naturally. Oils can also be tested for possible adulterants, contaminants and radioactivity. These procedures, however, are very costly.

An easy way to test the quality of an essential oil is to place a few drops on a piece of fabric or blotting paper. A quality essential oil will not leave a mark once it has evaporated, whereas if it has been diluted with oil it will leave a greasy stain. Pure essential oils are not greasy. Essential oils do have varying evaporation rates, so this test may take a while.

It is important to remember that the fragrance of an oil can change from season to season, due to varying conditions which can affect the plant source, as already discussed.

For aromatherapy purposes, it is important to be sure that the oil you purchase is from the correct botanical species, as not all species possess the therapeutic qualities required. All plants have a scientific name which identifies its own unique characteristics. These double names are universal; the first part refers to the genus or closely related group, while the second part of the name defines the type or species of the plant. To be sure that the oil you choose is indeed safe to use for aromatherapy, you can ask for it by the Latin name, which you will find indicated in the A–Z section. Also, if in doubt, check which part of the plant the oil has been extracted from as this too can make a difference. Juniper oil, for use in aromatherapy, should only come from the berries, for instance. There is a lower grade oil that is extracted from the twigs, but this is not recommended. If the supplier of the oil cannot tell you the Latin name and the part of the plant used, it is best to find one who can.

There are a number of tests that can be done to authenticate the quality of essential oils. As mentioned above, the problem is that these tests are expensive and must be performed on each new batch of essential oil. In 1987 the Natural Oils Research Association (NORA) was formed in the UK by Bernie Hephrun, who is the consultant to *The Aromatherapy Kit*, to formalize a procedure whereby oils could be tested and certified for quality. They devised the Aromark seal, which when found on the label of an essential oil ensures its quality and purity. Only natural products which have been produced by a single distillation or extraction process without anything being added can carry the Aromark seal. Products carrying the Aromark seal ensure that:

1. The essential oil is pure and has been derived from a named botanical species from a given origin.
2. It is a natural product which has been produced by a single distillation or extraction process.
3. The oil has been subjected to searching analytical procedures both at sampling and purchasing stages to establish its authenticity, composition and profile; and tested for any possible adulteration.
4. Batch numbers and identifications are issued and available from the supplier if not indicated on the specific bottle.

Not all pure essential oils carry the Aromark seal as yet, but it is rapidly becoming recognized as a mark of quality world-wide. Further information concerning the Aromark seal can be obtained from the Natural Oils Research Association (see Useful Addresses on page 111).

ESSENTIAL OILS VERSUS PERFUMES

Essential oils are the oldest form of perfume known. Originally they were used both for their scent and for their therapeutic qualities.

Today, perfumes are made up of a number of ingredients including:

- Aromatic oils – only good quality perfumes still use essential oils;
- Natural products of animal origin – ambergris, civet and musk – although these have now mostly been replaced by chemicals;
- Alcohol – used to dissolve the aromatic oils;
- Synthetic substances – designed to imitate the fragrance of naturally occurring scents. This is sometimes done by extracting certain constituents from essential oils and combining them with other substances.

Today's commercially prepared perfumes are used simply for their smell and have no therapeutic application, even when some constituents of essential oils are used. In order to have therapeutic effect, the whole structure must be present. Of course, it is possible to blend your own perfumes from essential oils (see chapter three).

Chapter 2

A–Z of Essential Oils

L isted in this chapter are the various plants from which we derive the main essential oils used in aromatherapy. For each one, the methods of distillation including the part of the plant used is indicated along with a brief synopsis of its history, major constituents, qualities and traditional uses. Cautions are indicated where applicable. These essential oils are safe to use as long as the guidelines in this book are followed. Some oils have a higher toxicity level than others which is why, in some cases, it is suggested that they only be used under the guidance of a qualified aromatherapist. It is for this reason that you will not find these oils listed in the chapters dealing with usage. Be sure to read the caution for each essential oil before using it; this together with the information on applying the oils provides complete details for safe usage. Only the main constituents contained in each essential oil are listed, as an essential oil can contain well over one hundred constituents.

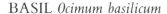

BASIL *Ocimum basilicum*
Top note; distilled from flowering tops and leaves

ORIGINS
Native to southern Asia and the Middle East. It is cultivated for commercial purposes in central and southern Europe, northern Africa, Asia and in subtropical America. In Italy the leaves are seen as a symbol of love because of their heart shape. Basil, which in Greek is short for 'basilikon phuton', means 'kingly herb'. *Ocimum* is derived from the Greek word meaning 'to smell', said to be named as a result of the pungent scent from the plants of this genus. It has been used in Chinese medicine for many centuries. Basil has traditionally been used in Hindu houses in India, where it is a sacred plant to Krishna and Vishnu, and is said to be the protecting spirit of the family.

MAIN CONSTITUENTS
Alcohol: linalol; ketones: borneone, camphor, cineole; phenols: methylchavicol, eugenol; terpenes: ocimene, pinene, sylvestrene.

QUALITIES
A refreshing, stimulating oil which makes an excellent nerve tonic; it strengthens concentration and clears the mind.

TRADITIONAL USES
A traditional remedy for chest infections, digestive problems, headaches and migraines. A good insect repellent.

CAUTIONS
Must be used in dilution as it can be irritating to sensitive skin. It can have an overstimulating effect but can also, when used excessively, cause grogginess. Avoid use during pregnancy.

BENZOIN (RESINOID)
Styrax benzoin
Base note; solvent extraction using gum-resin collected from bark of tree

ORIGINS
The benzoin tree is cultivated in Java, Sumatra, Cambodia, Vietnam, China and Thailand. The benzoin liquid is extracted by making an incision in the bark of the tree; the liquid is left to harden then collected. A resinoid is usually produced from the gum by mixing it with wood alcohol. A traditional ingredient in incense, benzoin fumes were thought to drive out evil spirits. Also known as 'balsam' and 'gum benjamin', although probably best known in 'Friar's Balsam' which is a compound tincture of benzoin for respiratory problems. Benzoin is commonly used as a fixative in perfumes.

MAIN CONSTITUENTS
Acids: benzoic, cinnamic; aldehyde: vanillin; ester: benzyl benzoate.

QUALITIES
A rich oil with a vanilla-like scent which contains anti-oxidative and preservative properties. Penetrating, warming and energizing.

TRADITIONAL USES
Helps with respiratory disorders and is particularly good used in inhalation for colds. Said to be effective for joint conditions such as gout and rheumatoid arthritis. Stimulates circulation.

Although Benzoin Resinoid is used by some aromatherapists it is not technically an essential oil, but a resin which is soluble in alcohol.

CAUTIONS
Excessive amounts could cause drowsiness.

BERGAMOT *Citrus bergamia*
*Top note; extracted by expression from
the rind of the fruit*

ORIGINS

The tree was first cultivated in Bergamo, Italy, from which its name derives. It is also grown commercially on the Ivory Coast. The fruit resembles a miniature orange with a greenish yellow colour when ripe. Italian folk medicine lists its use as primarily for fever and worms.

MAIN CONSTITUENTS

Alcohols: linalol, nerol, terpineol; ester: linalyl acetate; lactone: bergaptene★; terpenes: dipentene, limonene.
(★ Bergaptene is the constituent in Bergamot which causes photosensitization. There is, however, a standard of Bergamot oil which contains a percentage of bergaptene low enough to avoid this problem. This oil is known as Bergamot FCF, and it is the standard that is recommended for use in this book. FCF means Furo Coumarin Free.)

QUALITIES

Uplifting, delightful citrus scent. Powerful anti-depressant and nerve sedative. Excellent antiseptic qualities.

TRADITIONAL USES

Urinary tract infection, depression and anxiety. Also valuable in skin care. An effective deodorant and room fragrancer. Probably best known as a flavouring in Earl Grey tea and as one of the ingredients in eau-de-Cologne. A common ingredient in perfumes.

CAUTIONS

May be an irritant to sensitive skin. Should never be used neat as pigmentation may be effected. Should not be used on the skin (bath, perfume, etc.) prior to exposure to the sun as it increases photosensitivity. (Bergamot is sometimes used in sun tan preparations for this purpose; however, it is important to know that it does not protect the skin from burning.) Note that photosensitization cautions are not relevant if Bergamot FCF is used.

BLACK PEPPER *Piper nigrum*
Middle note; distilled from the fruit (peppercorn)

ORIGINS

One of the oldest known spices. Medicinal uses of black pepper were first described in a seventh-century herbal from the Tang Dynasty in China. Although pepper was used as a flavouring in food by the Romans and throughout the Middle Ages, it was also known as an appetite stimulant as well as an aid to digestion. The pepper plant is a native of south-western India but is also cultivated in Java, Sumatra and other tropical climates. The berries are picked from the plant just as they are beginning to turn red. They are then left to dry in the sun. Most of the essential oil is present in the skin of the berry.

MAIN CONSTITUENTS

Phenols: eugenol, myristicin, safrole; terpenes: bisabolene, camphene, farnesene, limonene, myrcene, phellandrene, pinene, sabinene, selinene, thujene; sesquiterpene: caryophyllene.

QUALITIES

A warming and invigorating oil; good for aches and pains. Stimulates circulation and digestion.

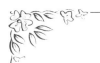
TRADITIONAL USES

Detoxifies by helping to remove phlegm from the body. Helpful in treating conditions of the gastro-intestinal tract. Increases appetite.

CAUTIONS

The proportion of Black Pepper used in a blend should be very low as it can cause skin irritation. Use in small quantities as a large dose may be damaging to the kidneys.

CAJEPUT *Melaleuca leucodendron*
Top note; distilled from the leaves and buds

ORIGINS

The name comes from the Malaysian 'kayu-puti' which means 'white wood'. Native to Australia, India and Malaysia and cultivated in tropical climates, particularly swamps. It was believed to be a panacea against skin diseases as well as stomach troubles.

MAIN CONSTITUENTS

Alcohol: terpineol; aldehyde: benzaldehyde; ketone: cineole; terpenes: dipentene, limonene, pinene.

QUALITIES

Very penetrating medicinal odour. Powerful stimulant.

TRADITIONAL USES

As an antiseptic in dentistry and the pharma-ceutical industry. It has also been traditionally used as a tea and as an insect repellent.

CAUTIONS

A powerful oil which should be used with care. Can be irritating to the skin and mucous membrane. It is recommended that this oil be used only under the direction of a qualified aromatherapist.

CAMPHOR *Cinnamomum camphora*
Middle note; distilled from the wood

ORIGINS

Camphor was traditionally used in China for embalming. It is grown in China, Borneo, Sri Lanka, Madagascar and other subtropical countries. Camphor can be found in every part of the tree but it is not extracted until the tree is at least 50 years old when it is hardy enough to withstand the necessary mutilation. Then it is removed by chipping off and boiling the wood in water. The camphor resin rises to the sur-face and becomes solid when the water cools. It can then be steam distilled in order to obtain the essential oil.

MAIN CONSTITUENTS

Alcohol: borneol; ketone: camphor; terpenes: camphene, pinene, dipentene.

QUALITIES

Has a balancing effect on the emotions making it useful in situations that cause imbalance such as shock. Powerful stimulant – to be used only in moderation.

TRADITIONAL USES

Stimulant for the heart, circulation as well as digestion. Used to raise low blood pressure. Preventative of infectious diseases. Used as an insecticide and as a moth repellent in the form of camphor balls.

CAUTIONS

Should not be used unless under the guidance

of a qualified aromatherapist. An excessive amount could cause convulsions and vomiting. In addition to being a skin irritant, it can act as a local circulatory irritant and numb peripheral sensory nerves. Not to be used if taking a homoeopathic remedy. Do not use if prone to epilepsy, asthma or high blood pressure. Avoid use during pregnancy.

CARAWAY *Carum carvi*
Top note; distilled from the seeds

ORIGINS
The plant from which caraway seeds come is native to Asia Minor and cultivated in northern Europe, Africa and Russia. It has been used in medicine as well as cooking since Egyptian times. Caraway was extensively used by the Romans in their cooking and was well known in Elizabethan England as both a flavouring and a digestive aid.

MAIN CONSTITUENTS
Aldehydes: acetaldehyde, cuminic, furfurol; ketone: carvone; terpene: limonene.

QUALITIES
Warming and stimulating. It is also an effective carminative.

TRADITIONAL USES
Flavouring in Kümmel liqueur. Over the years essential oil of Caraway has also been employed in perfumery and soap-making.

CAUTIONS
Recommended for use only under the guidance of a qualified aromatherapist. Can be irritating to sensitive skin types especially if used in concentration.

CEDARWOOD *Cedrus atlantica* or *Juniperus virginiana*
Base note; distilled from the wood of the tree

ORIGINS
The first known cedarwood (*Cedrus libani*) came from Lebanon and was used in Egypt for mummification and to make coffins. It was also considered a valuable ingredient in their medicine, cosmetics and perfumery. The wood was used to build the great Temple of Solomon in Jerusalem. *Cedrus atlantica*, a white cedarwood from Morocco, is considered to be closest in quality to *Cedrus libani* which is no longer available. *Juniperus virginiana*, also known as red cedarwood, comes from North America. The oils are thought to be similar in therapeutic action.

MAIN CONSTITUENTS
Alcohol: cedrol; sesquiterpenes: cadinene, cedrene, cedrenol.

QUALITIES
A mild, woody scent good for harmonizing and stabilizing unbalanced energies. It is mucolytic (breaks down mucus). Cedarwood is also a powerful antiseptic.

TRADITIONAL USES
As a remedy for cystitis and other urinary tract infections. Good for catarrhal conditions, particularly bronchitis. The wood was used to make storage chests as the odour of cedarwood repels moths and other insects. Also used as a fixative in perfumes.

CAUTIONS
High dosages may cause skin irritation. Do not use during pregnancy.

CHAMOMILE (ROMAN)
Anthemis nobilis
CHAMOMILE (GERMAN)
Matricaria chamomilla
Middle note; distilled from flowering tops

ORIGINS

The name 'chamomile' is derived from the Greek 'Kamai melon' which means 'ground apple', because the plant grows low on the ground and has an apple-like fragrance. Chamomile is one of the oldest herbs well known for its medicinal properties. Indeed, according to Nicholas Culpeper, chamomile was known to be effective for a wide range of complaints. It was also used in Egypt where it was thought to cure ague, a form of malaria. Roman (or wild) Chamomile is found in Britain and other parts of Europe and northern Africa, while German Chamomile grows in Germany as well as Hungary and Russia.

MAIN CONSTITUENTS

Roman Chamomile – acids: angelic, methacrylic, tiglic; sesquiterpenes: artemol, azulene★. German Chamomile – aldehyde: cuminic; sesquiterpene: azulene★.

(★ Azulene is formed as a result of the distillation process. German Chamomile contains more azulene than Roman Chamomile, hence its deep blue colour.)

QUALITIES

Best anti-inflammatory and anti-allergic oil. Good for aches and pains in both muscles and organs (earache, for example). Soothing and calming. Azulene has healing properties that act on scars. Chamomile has a low toxicity level, which makes it a safe oil to use on children as long as dosage recommendations are adhered to.

TRADITIONAL USES

For digestive disorders and insomnia. Used for liver, spleen and stomach complaints as well as general aches and pains. In shampoo for highlighting and conditioning blonde hair. Used as a tea to aid digestion and induce sleep.

CAUTIONS

Should not be used in the early months of pregnancy. Most effective in small dosages.

CINNAMON LEAF
Cinnamomum zeylanicum
Base note; distilled from leaves

ORIGINS

Native to Sri Lanka and cultivated in India, Jamaica, Brazil, the Seychelles and other tropical countries. Considered by the ancients to be one of the most important aromatic spices. Legend has it that it was given to King Solomon by the Queen of Sheba and was one of the spices used to anoint the Ark of the Covenant, which contained the scrolls of Jewish holy law.

MAIN CONSTITUENTS

Alcohol: linalol; aldehydes: benzaldehyde, cinnamic, furfurol; phenols: eugenol, safrole; terpenes: cymene, dipentene, phellandrene, pinene.

QUALITIES

A rich, spicy, warming oil with an uplifting fragrance that soothes nausea. Stimulates circulation and digestion. A strong antiseptic.

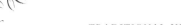
TRADITIONAL USES

For flavouring in foods and drink. An ingredient in some dental products.

CAUTIONS

A powerful oil which should be used with care and only in small amounts. Avoid use during pregnancy.

CLARY SAGE *Salvia sclarea*
Middle note (sometimes top); distilled from leaves and flowering tops

ORIGINS

It is believed that 'clary' is derived from the Latin, '*clarus*', which means 'clear'. It was called 'Clear Eye' in the Middle Ages as it was known for its ability to heal eye problems. It was sometimes used as a substitute for hops in Britain because of its intoxicating property. In Germany it was known as 'Muskatel Salbei' and was used to adulterate wine. Native to Italy, Syria, southern France and Switzerland. Also cultivated in other locations with dry soil such as Morocco.

MAIN CONSTITUENTS

Alcohols: linalol, salviol; ester: linalyl acetate; ketone: cineole; sesquiterpene: caryophyllene; terpenes: pinene, myrcene, phellandrene.

QUALITIES

A euphoric, warming and very powerful relaxant. A good tonic.

TRADITIONAL USES

For stressful and tense situations. Used to combat night sweats resulting from tuberculosis. Sometimes used in the production of muscatel wine.

CAUTIONS

Do not use Clary Sage when alcohol has been consumed. It should not be used when alertness is required (for example, in a massage before having to drive) because it can cause drowsiness. Use sparingly as large doses can cause contra-indications (in small doses Clary Sage is mildly hypotensive; however, if large amounts are used the opposite effect can occur). Avoid use during pregnancy.

CLOVE BUD *Eugenia caryophyllata*
Base note; distilled from the flower buds

ORIGINS

Native to south-east Asia. Used in China during the Han Dynasty in the third century BC as a breath sweetener as well as for the relief of toothache. One of the spices known and extensively used by the Romans.

MAIN CONSTITUENTS

Aldehyde: furfurol; ester: methyl salicylate; phenol: eugenol; sesquiterpene: caryophyllene; terpene: pinene.

QUALITIES

Warming, spicy tonic. A powerful antiseptic, which makes it useful for all kinds of infection; also a known carminative.

TRADITIONAL USES

A well-known toothache remedy. Also used in the past to soothe stomach upsets. Used as a food flavouring agent.

CAUTIONS

A very powerful oil which should be used with care. Not suggested for use as a massage oil as it can be highly irritating to the skin.

CORIANDER *Coriandrum sativum*
Top note; distilled from the seeds

ORIGINS
Cultivated world-wide, it has been known for over 3000 years having been mentioned by early Sanskrit writers. Coriander seeds were discovered in Egyptian tombs. Its name is derived from 'koris', which is Greek for 'bed-bug', and it seems the plant smells strongly of these insects. Fortunately, the seeds do not carry this same odour.

MAIN CONSTITUENTS
Alcohols: borneol, geraniol, linalol, terpineol; ketone: cineole; terpenes: cymene, dipentene, phellandrene, pinene, terpinene, terpinolene.

QUALITIES
A warming and stimulating oil.

TRADITIONAL USES
The seeds are chewed to stimulate secretion of gastric juices. An ingredient of the liqueurs Chartreuse and Benedictine.

CAUTIONS
Can cause drowsiness in large doses.

CYPRESS *Cupressus sempervirens*
Middle/base note; distilled from leaves and cones

ORIGINS
The Egyptians associated the tree with death; *sempervirens* means 'ever lasting' which ironically connects it to the Egyptian belief in the afterlife. Cypress trees are very often found in cemeteries, especially in the Mediterranean region to which they are native. Cypress has been used as a purification incense by the Tibetans.

MAIN CONSTITUENTS
Alcohol: sabinol; aldehyde; furfurol; ester: terpenyl acetate; terpenes: camphene, cymene, pinene, sylvestrene.

QUALITIES
A resinous, woody oil. Very astringent and uniquely useful in cases of excessive fluid discharges. Soothing and refreshing.

TRADITIONAL USES
Helpful with varicose veins and haemorrhoids. An ingredient used to treat whooping cough. Used in men's aftershave lotion and in deodorant. Often employed as an insect repellent.

CAUTIONS
Avoid use during pregnancy. Do not massage directly on varicose veins.

EUCALYPTUS
(See chapter seven)

FENNEL (SWEET) *Foeniculum vulgare*
Middle note; distilled from the crushed seeds

ORIGINS
Fennel grows wild in most parts of Europe. The Romans believed that it helped to promote good vision as well as being a cure for obesity. In China, according to a sixth-century herbal, it was used to restore flavour to meat that had gone off. In mediaeval times it was used as a protection against evil influences.

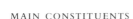

MAIN CONSTITUENTS

Aldehydes: anisic, cuminic; phenols: anethole, methylchavicol; terpenes: camphene, dipentene, limonene, phellandrene.

QUALITIES

Excellent carminative, good for digestion. Also a useful diuretic.

TRADITIONAL USES

Used for cellulitis and obesity. Fennel was thought to be an antidote for snake bites and poisonous plants. Also used to counterbalance alcohol poisoning.

CAUTIONS

Not to be used on young children or people with epilepsy. Can cause skin irritation in sensitive individuals.

FRANKINCENSE *Boswellia thurifera* or *Boswellia carteri*
Base note; distilled from tree resin

ORIGINS

The name Frankincense derives from mediaeval French meaning 'luxuriant incense'. However, this name was given to the plant in the tenth century: its original name is Olibanum, the term most professional aromatherapists still use. It is believed that the name Olibanum derives from 'oil from Lebanon' as it is native to the Middle East. The resin is collected from the tree by cutting into the trunk and allowing it to exude and harden. Its earliest known use, dating back some 5000 years, was as incense. It was used by the Egyptians in their temple rituals and to rejuvenate the skin.

MAIN CONSTITUENTS

Alcohol: olibanol; sesquiterpene: cadinene; terpenes: camphene, dipentene, pinene, phellandrene.

QUALITIES

A warm, spicy oil which is comforting for states of anxiety. Used in vaporization to deepen breathing. A useful aid for meditation.

TRADITIONAL USES

For meditation and relaxation. Used for respiratory infections and to fumigate sick rooms. Also used to rejuvenate the skin.

GERANIUM
(See chapter seven)

GINGER *Zingiber officinale*
Base note; distilled from roots

ORIGINS

Used in Chinese medicine to cope with excessive moisture in the body. One of the first oriental spices to reach the West, used both in cooking and for its medicinal properties. It was used as a remedy against the plague and in pomanders to dispel odours. In cooking it is considered an aid for digestion. Native to Asia and cultivated in tropical climates.

MAIN CONSTITUENTS

Alcohol: borneol; aldehyde: citral; ketone: cineole; sesquiterpene: zingiberene; terpenes: camphene, limonene, phellandrene.

QUALITIES

A tangy, rich oil. Stimulating general tonic.

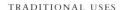

TRADITIONAL USES

Appetite stimulant. Used in cooking and as an aid against travel sickness. Stimulant for the circulatory system.

CAUTIONS

Can be irritating to the skin. Avoid use during pregnancy.

HYSSOP *Hyssopus officinalis*
Middle note; distilled from flowering tops

ORIGINS

Native to the Mediterranean region. Regarded by the Greeks and Hebrews as a sacred herb, it was used to cleanse sacred areas such as temples.

MAIN CONSTITUENTS

Alcohols: borneol, linalol; ketones: camphor, pinocamphone, thujone; sesquiterpene: candinene; terpenes: camphene, pinene.

QUALITIES

Useful for chest infections, particularly catarrh. Also helps cuts and bruises.

TRADITIONAL USES

A disinfectant. An ingredient in the liqueur Chartreuse.

CAUTIONS

Hyssop contains a high percentage of ketones which can make it somewhat toxic and so there are a number of conditions, including pregnancy, high blood pressure and epilepsy, for which it should not be used. For this reason it is best to use this oil only under the guidance of a qualified aromatherapist.

JASMINE *Jasminum officinale* or *Jasminum grandiflorum*
Base note; usually extracted by volatile solvents from the flowers

ORIGINS

Considered the 'king of oils', it is native to the Himalayas and cultivated in China, India, France and the Mediterranean region. The flowers are strung in garlands and presented to honoured guests by Hindus. Blooms are harvested at night when, due to chemical action, the fragrance is strongest.

MAIN CONSTITUENTS

Alcohols: benzyl, farnesol, geraniol, linalol, nerol, terpineol; esters: linalyl acetate, methyl anthranilate; ketone: jasmone; phenol: eugenol.

QUALITIES

Excellent anti-depressant, aphrodisiac and strong sensual stimulant.

TRADITIONAL USES

To scent tea. As an aphrodisiac. To ease labour during childbirth. In the cosmetic industry.

CAUTIONS

If used in excess, Jasmine can cause contra-indications. Should not be used in the early stages of pregnancy.

JUNIPER BERRY *Juniperus communis*
Middle note; distilled from dried fruits

ORIGINS

Found in many places in the northern hemisphere, the essential oil is produced mainly in Hungary. Used in antiquity both as incense to keep away evil spirits and as a disinfectant during times of plague. The Egyptians, as part of the embalming process, rubbed the oil along with other ingredients, on the body to help make it supple. They also used Juniper berries for a variety of medical purposes including flatulence and indigestion. More recently juniper sprigs were burnt in hospital wards in France to protect against infection. The oil was used in body massage against fever and smallpox.

MAIN CONSTITUENTS

Alcohols: borneol, terpineol; sesquiterpenes: caryophyllene, cadinene, elemene; terpenes: camphene, pinene, limonene, mercene, sabinene.

QUALITIES

A refreshing and invigorating oil. It has antiseptic, astringent and diuretic properties. Detoxifying and cleansing.

TRADITIONAL USES

Urinary, respiratory and gastro-intestinal infections. An ingredient in gin.

CAUTIONS

Avoid use during pregnancy. When used excessively it can cause inflammation to the kidneys and urine retention.

LAVENDER
(See chapter eight)

LEMON *Citrus limomum*
Top note; expression from the rind of the fruit

ORIGINS

Originally from Persia, the tree spread throughout the Mediterranean. Contains citric acid and according to Mrs Grieve in *A Modern Herbal*,

'English ships are required by law to carry sufficient lemon or lime juice for every seaman to have an ounce daily after being ten days at sea'. This was to protect them from scurvy.

MAIN CONSTITUENTS

Alcohol: linalol; aldehydes: citral, citronellal; ester: geraniol; sesquiterpene: cadinene; terpenes: bisabolene, camphene, dipentene, limonene, pinene, phellandrene.

QUALITIES

A refreshing, cleansing light oil. Excellent antiseptic and disinfectant.

TRADITIONAL USES

By the drug industry as an ingredient in cold and flu remedies. Classic remedy for sore throats. Used extensively in cooking.

CAUTIONS

Should only be used in small amounts. May cause skin irritation.

LEMONGRASS *Cymbopogon citratus*
Top note; distilled from the grass

ORIGINS

Grows wild in Malaysia and is cultivated in the West Indies, Brazil and other tropical climates. Used in traditional Indian medicine for infectious illnesses and to reduce fevers.

MAIN CONSTITUENTS

Alcohols: farnesol, geraniol, nerol; aldehydes: citral, citronellal; terpenes: limonene, myrcene.

QUALITIES

An invigorating oil. Antiseptic and antibacterial qualities. A gastric stimulant.

TRADITIONAL USES

In cooking. As an insect repellent and as an

ingredient to help protect animals from fleas and tics. Lemongrass has long been used in traditional Indian medicine to fight infectious illnesses and fevers. Sometimes used to adulterate Melissa or Verbena essential oils which are both more expensive.

CAUTIONS
Use in low dosages. Can be irritating to sensitive skin.

MANDARIN *Citrus nobilis*
or *Citrus madurensis*
or *Citrus reticulata*
Top note; expressed from the peel
ORIGINS
Mandarin oranges were introduced to Europe in the nineteenth century. Considered to be an oil of joy, it is one of the few oils, along with Lavender, that is safe to use on children. In France it is used as a remedy for stomach upsets in children.

MAIN CONSTITUENTS
Alcohol: geraniol; aldehydes: citral, citronellal; ester: methyl anthranilate; terpene: limonene.

QUALITIES
An appealing, sweet oil with an almost floral citrus scent. It is stimulating in a gentle way, which makes it an excellent oil for the liver and digestive function in elderly individuals.

TRADITIONAL USES
Ingredient in fruit compotes and drinks. Also used in soaps, cosmetics and perfumes.

MARJORAM *Origanum majorana*
or *Thymus mastichina*
Middle note; distilled from flowering tops
ORIGINS
Native to the Mediterranean region. *Majorana* in Latin means 'major' and the herb was thought to convey long life. Marjoram was used by the Ancient Greeks: the word *origanum* comes from two Greek words, 'oros' for mountain and 'ganos' which means joy. It is closely linked to Oregano. *Thymus mastichina*, another species of marjoram, is from Spain.

MAIN CONSTITUENTS
Alcohols: borneol, terpineol; ketone: camphor; sesquiterpene: caryophyllene; terpenes: pinene, sabinene, terpinene.

QUALITIES
A warming oil for both body and mind. Stimulating. A useful emmenagogue.

TRADITIONAL USES
As a common kitchen herb and tea. In Germany it is called 'wurstkraut' (sausage herb), as it is used as a flavouring in meats. Used to combat menstrual problems.

CAUTIONS
Excessive use can cause drowsiness, dull the senses and deaden the emotions. Because of this, it is sometimes considered to be an anti-aphrodisiac. Avoid use during pregnancy.

MELISSA *Melissa officinalis*
Middle note; distilled from the leaves and tops
ORIGINS
Native to Europe, middle Asia and North America, it is often referred to as 'lemon

balm'. It was known in Greece as 'melissophyllon' which is Greek for 'bee leaf' as indeed bees are very attracted to the plant.

MAIN CONSTITUENTS

Acid: citronellic; alcohols: citrolellol, geraniol, linalol; aldehydes: citral, citronellal; ester: geranyl; sesquiterpene: caryophyllene.

QUALITIES

This oil has a light rejuvenating scent with anti-depressant and anti-spasmodic properties. It calms and releases tension, generating an uplifting and joyful effect. It can be very soothing if used in times of shock or bereavement.

TRADITIONAL USES

As a tea, in distilling liqueurs (Benedictine and Chartreuse) and in cooking. A valuable insect repellent.

CAUTIONS

Can be irritating to the skin. Avoid use during pregnancy.

MYRRH *Commiphora myrrha*
Base note; distilled from the resin

ORIGINS

The name is believed to be derived from the old Hebrew and Arabic word 'mur' which means 'bitter'. Native to northern Africa and Asia, it requires very dry conditions for growth. The resin is secreted either naturally or when the bark is cut. It is closely related to Frankincense. Known from antiquity in incense, perfumes and medicine as well as being one of the ingredients the Egyptians used for embalming.

MAIN CONSTITUENTS

Acid: myrrholic; aldehydes: cinnamic, cuminic; phenol: eugenol; sesquiterpene: cadinene; terpenes: dipentene, heerabolene, limonene, pinene.

QUALITIES

A rich, amber oil with strong healing, antiseptic and rejuvenating properties. An expectorant and anti-inflammatory.

TRADITIONAL USES

In healing ointments. As an ingredient in toothpaste and mouthwash.

CAUTIONS

Relatively mild oil, but advisable to avoid use during pregnancy.

NEROLI *Citrus aurantium*
Base note; extracted by enfleurage and sometimes distilled from orange blossoms

ORIGINS

The essential oil from Tunisia, Italy and North America. There are a number of suggestions as to where the name 'Neroli' came from. Some say that it takes its name from the sixteenth-century Italian Princess Anne-Marie of Nerola because she used it as her perfume. It has also been suggested that the name comes from the Emperor Nero. It is interesting that, according to Mrs Grieve, both the common and official name for this plant come from the Sanskrit 'nagaranga' ('naranj' in Arabic). Orange flower water is a by-product of the distillation process.

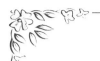

MAIN CONSTITUENTS

Acid: phenylacetic; alcohols: nerol, geraniol, linalol, nerolidol, terpineol; esters: linalyl acetate, methyl anthranilate, neryl acetate; ketone: jasmone; terpenes: camphene, limonene.

QUALITIES

An exquisite, intoxicating scent. Calms the emotions. Anti-depressant, antiseptic and aphrodisiac.

TRADITIONAL USES

One of the main ingredients in eau-de-Cologne. Used as a flavouring agent and in the perfume industry. The blossoms are used in bridal wreaths.

CAUTIONS

A mildly sedative oil, so should not be used when alertness is necessary.

NIAOULI *Melaleuca viridiflora*
Top note; distilled from the leaves and young twigs of the Niaouli plant

ORIGINS

Originally known as Gomenol, as it was first distilled and shipped from Gomen in the French East Indies. *Melaleuca* refers to 'old and new bark', as 'melos' is 'black' and 'leucos' is 'white' in Greek. Used in hospital wards in France, because of its antiseptic properties.

MAIN CONSTITUENTS

Acid: valeric; alcohol: terpineol; ketone: cineole; terpenes: limonene, pinene.

QUALITIES

Powerful antiseptic and tissue stimulant, therefore helpful in healing wounds and burns.

TRADITIONAL USES

Used in pharmaceutical preparations such as gargles and mouth sprays.

NUTMEG *Myristica fragrans*
Base note; distilled from the seeds

ORIGINS

Native to the Far East and cultivated in tropical climates. Its use in China dates back to around the fifth century and was considered to be beneficial for the spleen, stomach and large intestine. One of several fumigant aromatics used in the streets of Rome during the coronation of Emperor Henry VI. It has long been recognized that, when used in moderation, Nutmeg can produce hallucinations. These are caused by myristicin, one of its constituents (see below), and a psychotropic (a substance which has an effect on moods) not too dissimilar from mescaline, which is found in the Peyote Cactus.

MAIN CONSTITUENTS

Alcohols: borneol, geraniol, linalol, terpineol; phenols: eugenol, myristicin, safrol; terpenes: camphene, dipentene, pinene.

QUALITIES

A rich, spicy and warming oil. Very stimulating.

TRADITIONAL USES

A flavouring in foods and drinks. An ingredient in some hair lotions and dental products.

CAUTIONS

A powerful oil which should be used with care; excessive amounts can cause mental or nervous disturbances. Therefore, it is recommended for use only under the guidance of a qualified aromatherapist. Can be irritating to the skin. Avoid use during pregnancy.

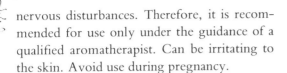

ORANGE *Citrus aurantium*
Top note; extracted from the peel

ORIGINS
Native to the Far East and cultivated in the Mediterranean, Israel and North and South America. Considered to be the 'golden apple' which is referred to in Greek mythology.

MAIN CONSTITUENTS
Alcohol: nerol; aldehydes: citral, citronellal; ester: methyl anthranilate; terpene: limonene.

QUALITIES
A delicious sweet scent. Sedative. A lovely room freshener in vaporization.

TRADITIONAL USES
Both in the perfume and food industry. An ingredient of the liqueur Curaçao.

CAUTIONS
Excessive use can cause skin irritation.

PATCHOULI *Pogostemon patchouli*
Base note; distilled from the leaves

ORIGINS
Native to south-east Asia and India. It is used as a scent for Indian linen, making it easy to recognize. It is cultivated in subtropical climates. Was used as an antidote for poisonous snake bites. Very popular during the 1960s 'flower power' era.

MAIN CONSTITUENTS
Alcohol: patchoulol; aldehydes: benzoic, cinnamic; phenol: eugenol; sesquiterpenes: cadinene, patchoulene.

QUALITIES
A musky, sweet, sensual oil, which is renowned as an aphrodisiac. Stimulating. Pungent – making it a good masking scent to override unwanted smells, although many people find the smell of Patchouli offensive in itself.

TRADITIONAL USES
As a fixative in perfumes and incense. An ingredient in genuine Indian shawls as well as Indian ink. Used to mask other odours.

CAUTIONS
Can be sedative in low doses and stimulating when used in excess. Can cause loss of appetite.

PEPPERMINT *Mentha piperita*
Middle note; distilled from leaves and flowering tops

ORIGINS
Native to Europe but cultivated widely including North America and Japan. It was first recorded in England in the early part of the seventeenth century by both Gerard and Culpeper. Used by Greek physicians and may well have been known by the Egyptians.

MAIN CONSTITUENTS
Alcohols: amyl, menthol; ester: menthyl acetate; ketones: carvone, cineole, jasmone, menthone; phenol: carvacrol; sesquiterpene: cadinene; terpenes: limonene, phellandrene.

QUALITIES

A cooling and invigorating oil, which has a warming effect too.

TRADITIONAL USES

An ingredient in toothpaste and cosmetics, as well as cough, cold and digestive remedies. Popular flavouring in confectionery. Often used for insect and vermin control.

CAUTIONS

Not to be used excessively. Can be an irritant to mucous membranes and the skin. Avoid use during pregnancy and while breastfeeding as it could discourage milk flow. Should not be used when taking homoeopathic remedies.

PETITGRAIN *Citrus aurantium*
Top note; distilled from leaves of the bitter orange tree

ORIGINS

Native to the Far East and cultivated in France, Tunisia, Italy and North America. The name means 'small grain'. Originally the oil came from the unripe fruit; however, because it reduced the mature orange crop drastically, the leaves, sometimes mixed with twigs, began to be used.

MAIN CONSTITUENTS

Alcohols: farnesol, geraniol, linalol, nerol, nerolidol, terpineol; aldehyde: citral; esters: geranyl acetate, linalyl acetate; terpenes: camphene, limonene.

QUALITIES

Similar properties to Neroli, but less refined in fragrance and less sedative. Excellent fixative in massage blends and perfumes.

TRADITIONAL USES

Sometimes used in place of Neroli (it comes from the same plant) often due to the cost difference. A flavouring in foods and drinks.

PINE NEEDLE *Abies sibirica*
Middle note; distilled from the needles and cones

ORIGINS

Pine Needle essential oil is obtained from the Norwegian Pine. The resin produced from the trunk of many species of pine tree is used to produce Turpentine oil, a solvent which is mainly used in varnishes and oil-based paints.

MAIN CONSTITUENTS

Alcohol: borneol; esters: bornyl acetate, terpinyl acetate; sesquiterpene: cadinene; terpenes: camphene, dipentene, phellandrene, pinene, sylvestrene.

QUALITIES

A pungent, clean scent. Powerful antiseptic.

TRADITIONAL USES

Often found as an ingredient in disinfectants, cleaning agents and room deodorizers.

CAUTIONS

Can be irritating to the skin.

ROSE ABSOLUTE *Rosa centifolia* and ROSE OTTO *Rosa damascena*
Base note; Absolute extracted with solvents; Otto steam distilled from the petals

ORIGINS

The flower is known in many countries;

however, the oil is mainly obtained from Bulgaria, France, Morocco and Turkey. It is considered to be the 'queen of essential oils'. '*Centifolia*' means 'one hundred petals'. In alchemy the rose symbolizes mystical or divine love and it is believed that the tenth-century alchemist, Avicenna, was the first to produce a distillation from the flower. Venus is said to have coloured the rose with her blood when Adonis was killed by a boar. Rose Otto, the finest of the Rose oils, is from Bulgaria and it takes about thirty roses to make one drop of this oil. Rose petals were scattered at weddings to ensure a happy marriage and today's use of confetti could well be linked to this custom.

MAIN CONSTITUENTS
For both Rose oils – acid: geranic; alcohols: citronnellol, geraniol, farnesol, nerol; phenol: eugenol; terpene: myrcene.

QUALITIES
A beautiful, feminine scent. One of the most antiseptic essences and least toxic essential oils. Powerful anti-depressant. The best remedy for treating disorders of the feminine reproductive system.

TRADITIONAL USES
Widely used in the cosmetic industry. Also used in food preparation (especially Persian) as a flavouring agent, particularly in the form of rosewater.

CAUTIONS
Avoid use during pregnancy.

ROSEMARY
(See chapter seven)

ROSEWOOD *Aniba rosaeodora*
Middle note; distilled from the wood chippings

ORIGINS
The tree grows in the Amazon rainforest, although most of the essential oil is obtained from Guyana because of the controversy of felling in the rainforest. Rosewood is a protected species in Brazil.

MAIN CONSTITUENTS
Alcohols: geraniol, linalol, nerol, terpineol; ketone: cineole; terpene: dipentene.

QUALITIES
An excellent room freshener and ideal to blend with other aromas for skin care and perfume.

TRADITIONAL USES
Used by the cosmetic industry in bath and skin care products.

SAGE *Salvia officinalis*
Top note; distilled from leaves and flowers

ORIGINS
There are many species of sage which are widely distributed throughout the world, having various uses from culinary to hallucinogenic. *Salvia officinalis* is the most important and has been cultivated for thousands of years. It is native to southern Europe. *Salvia* comes from the Latin word which means 'I save'. The Romans called it 'herba sacra' which means 'sacred herb'.

MAIN CONSTITUENTS
Alcohols: borneol, salvio; ketones: camphor, cineole, thujone; terpene: phellandrene.

QUALITIES

An extremely stimulating essential oil.

TRADITIONAL USES

Used widely in cooking. Used medicinally in gargles and poultices.

CAUTIONS

As the essential oil contains a high proportion of the ketone thujone, which can provoke epileptic fits and convulsions, and can be toxic if taken in excess, it is recommended for use only under the guidance of a qualified aromatherapist.

SANDALWOOD *Santalum album*
Base note; distilled from the heart of the wood

ORIGINS

The best quality essential oil comes from the Sandalwood grown in Mysore in southern India. The tree is cut when it is mature and close to its demise. Only the heart of the wood is used to distil the oil. Used in *Ayurveda*, the Indian system of healing, for a number of complaints including acne, poisonous stings and external bleeding, as well as being used as a blood purifier and in massage.

MAIN CONSTITUENTS

Alcohol: santalol; aldehyde: furfurol; sesquiterpene: santalene.

QUALITIES

A sweet, woody scent which evokes a meditative atmosphere. Useful for states of anxiety and nervous tension.

TRADITIONAL USES

Used as an ingredient in perfumes, soaps and cosmetics. A popular ingredient for incense.

TAGETES *Tagetes glandulifera*
Base note; distilled from the leaves and flowers

ORIGINS

Grows in South America, Mexico, Africa, Asia and Europe as well as North America. Sometimes known as African Marigold but should not be confused with Calendula. Used in southern Chinese medicine to alleviate fever, treat colds and disperse phlegm.

MAIN CONSTITUENTS

Ketone: tagetone; terpenes: limonene, ocimene.

QUALITIES

Fruity fragrance with fungicidal properties.

TRADITIONAL USES

In India it is a popular ingredient in perfumes.

CAUTIONS

A powerful oil which should only be used under the guidance of a qualified practitioner. Can cause skin irritation.

TARRAGON *Artemisia dracunculus*
Base note; distilled from the leaves

ORIGINS

Native to southern Europe. Was used as an antidote for snake bites. Its name may be derived from the Latin 'dracunculus', which means 'little dragon'.

MAIN CONSTITUENTS

Phenol: methylchavicol; terpenes: ocimene, phellandrene.

QUALITIES

A warming and stimulating essential oil.

TRADITIONAL USES

A popular ingredient in French cuisine and said to be stimulating to the appetite.

CAUTIONS

Use only under the guidance of a qualified practitioner. Do not use during pregnancy.

TEA TREE
(See chapter seven)

THYME *Thymus vulgaris*
Top note; distilled from the flowering tops

ORIGINS

The word derives from the Greek 'thymos' which means 'to perfume'. Native to the Mediterranean region, it is cultivated in many countries including China, Germany and Hungary. The essential oil was first isolated in Germany in the early eighteenth century and used for its powerful antiseptic quality.

MAIN CONSTITUENTS

Alcohols: borneol, linalol; phenols: carvacrol, thymol; sesquiterpene: caryophyllene; terpenes: cymene, terpinene.

QUALITIES

A very powerful, antiseptic oil. Strengthening and invigorating for physical and mental debility of all kinds. In vaporization it combats infectious diseases.

TRADITIONAL USES

Used extensively in cooking. An ingredient in toothpaste and mouthwash. A very powerful disinfectant. Extensively used in both the food and drink industries.

CAUTIONS

Should only be used under the guidance of a qualified practitioner. Best not to use in the bath or as a massage oil as it could be irritating to the skin and mucous membranes. Do not use if high blood pressure is a problem. Avoid use during pregnancy.

YLANG YLANG *Cananga odorata*
Base note; distilled from the flowers

ORIGINS

The name means 'flower of flowers' and it is grown in the Philippines, Comores, Java, Sumatra and Madagascar. There are a number of grades of oil, the best comes from the first phase of distillation as it has the finer perfume.

MAIN CONSTITUENTS

Acid: benzoic; alcohols: farnesol, geraniol, linalol; ester: benzyl acetate; phenols: eugenol, safrol, ylangol; sesquiterpene: cadinene; terpene; pinene.

QUALITIES

A very sweet exotic scent, which makes an interesting perfume in its own right. It is a reputed aphrodisiac, a powerful sensual stimulant and euphoric. It has a sedative and regulating effect on the nervous system.

TRADITIONAL USES

An ingredient of Macassar hair oil, which was used on the scalp to encourage hair growth, popular in the nineteenth century. Ylang Ylang is widely used in the cosmetic industry as a fragrance component.

CAUTIONS

Not to be used in concentrated amounts as excessive use could cause headaches and nausea. Could be an irritant to sensitive skin.

Chapter 3

USING ESSENTIAL OILS

Aromatherapy can be beneficial to almost everyone. And, as we shall see in this chapter, there are many ways that most of the oils can be used safely in treatments at home. These range from massage, probably the most well-known method of treatment, to aromatherapy baths, creams and vaporizers, all of which are described fully in this chapter. If you have ever contemplated visiting a professional aromatherapist for treatment, you will learn what to expect in the following pages. Before you begin to experiment with your oils, however, please read the opening section of this chapter, which outlines the warnings concerning the use of essential oils and suggests some precautions you should take before applying oils to the skin. It is important to remember that when dealing with serious or specific complaints, it is advisable to consult a qualified medical practitioner.

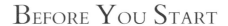

Before You Start

Essential oils are highly concentrated, as already discussed in chapter one, and therefore must be used and stored with great care. Before attempting to use your essential oils in any of the treatments suggested in this chapter, it is important that you are aware of any contra-indications that might occur as a result of their use. Certain oils can be potentially dangerous when used in particular situations, such as pregnancy, and others can cause skin irritations. It is vital therefore, that you read the warnings given on the following pages. All applications are for external use only; essential oils should only be taken internally under the direction of a qualified aromatherapist.

SKIN SENSITIVITY

When using essential oils for the first time, it is always best to use small amounts, as some may be irritating to certain skin types. The amount can then be increased to the maximum recommended for future applications.

Generally, though by no means a firm rule, fair-haired people have sensitive skin. They tend to burn easily in the sun and their skin is very delicate looking. It will redden quickly, sometimes just by coming into contact with tight clothing or elastic on sleeves. If you are planning to apply the essential oils directly to the skin by using a massage blend, it may be a good idea to pre-test the blend on a small area of skin beforehand. It is also best to start with the gentle oils, such as Chamomile, Lavender,

USE OF ESSENTIAL OILS WHICH ARE POTENTIAL SKIN IRRITANTS

Essential oil	Maximum percentage of essential oil in blend	Max. no. of essential oil drops in the bath
Basil	1%	2
Black Pepper	1%	2
Cinnamon Leaf	<1%	1
Clary Sage	1%	2
Clove Bud	<1%	0
Fennel	1%	2
Grapefruit	1%	2
Ginger	1%	2
Jasmine	1%	2
Juniper	1%	3
Lemon	1%	3
Lemongrass	1%	3
Melissa	1%	3
Nutmeg	1%	2
Orange	1%	4
Peppermint	<1%	1
Pine	1%	2

Notes
- 2 drops of essential oil per 10 ml of dilutant is the equivalent of a 1% blend.
- For other applications (local wash, foot-bath, etc.) use only 1 drop of essential oils listed on this chart.

< *means less than a 1% blend.*

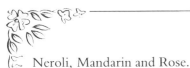

Neroli, Mandarin and Rose.

There are a few essential oils that can cause a severe skin reaction when exposed to sunlight (photosensitivity). Bergamot, in particular, can be a problem as discussed previously (see page 28). It is advisable to use Bergamot FCF from which the main constituent which causes the sensitivity, bergaptene, has been removed. There are other essential oils, such as Mandarin, Orange and Lemon that have constituents which can cause photosensitivity, but the percentages of these constituents are so low that the recommended dosages for these essential oils as indicated in this book should not cause problems.

Essential oils should be diluted in either whole milk or grapeseed oil before dispersing in the bath. It is also best to use about half the recommended amount in massage blends. This means about 2 drops of essential oil for every 10 ml of carrier oil. A light carrier oil such as grapeseed is recommended.

A number of oils should only be used in small amounts because they can be potential skin irritants. It is therefore suggested that people with sensitive skin avoid these oils altogether unless under the instructions of a qualified therapist. Oils that should be diluted before use are shown in the chart opposite.

PREGNANCY

A number of oils stimulate menstruation (emmenagogues) and should be avoided at least during the first few months of pregnancy. These oils include Basil, Chamomile, Clary Sage, Cypress, Fennel, Hyssop, Juniper, Lavender, Marjoram, Myrrh, Peppermint, Rose and Rosemary. As a general rule, it is best to use only essential oils from flowers, woods or citrus during pregnancy, avoiding completely essential oils derived from herbs. However, it is always a good idea to check with a qualified aromatherapist if you are not totally sure, particularly during the first few months. Many aromatherapists feel that Chamomile and Lavender, although classified as emmenagogues, can be used with moderation even at the beginning of a pregnancy unless there is reason to believe that a risk of miscarriage exists.

There are a number of ways that essential oils can be beneficial during pregnancy so rather than being afraid to use them at all, it is well worth getting guidance from a qualified practitioner. For example, lower back pain is a common complaint during pregnancy because of the increased weight and reshaping of the body. Massage with essential oils can offer much relief during this time.

AROMATHERAPY TREATMENT FOR CHILDREN AND THE ELDERLY

Some essential oils, Chamomile, Lavender or Mandarin being the best choices, are safe to use on children provided a few simple precautions are taken. The essential oil must always be diluted first, even before putting into the bath water. This can easily be done by placing 1 drop of the essential oil into a few teaspoons of either almond oil or whole milk. Be sure that the blend is mixed well before dispersing it into the bath water. This is especially true for infants as they usually suck their thumb or other parts of the hand, rub their eyes, etc. As oil and water do not readily mix, this oil can find its way onto the infant's hand which can, just as quickly find its way into the mouth. Always keep the essential oils, diluted and otherwise, away from the eye area. This, of course, is true for adults as well.

When preparing a massage blend for children, use about half the amount of essential oil you would for an adult: 2 drops of essential oil to 10 ml almond oil is about right.

Of course, you should never try to treat a serious illness yourself without the guidance of a professional therapist.

It is generally safe to use essential oil on the elderly as long as the guidelines outlined in this book are followed. When using them in the bath, it is probably best to dilute essential oils first (see above).

STORAGE AND CARE OF ESSENTIAL OILS

Essential oils are susceptible to the effects of heat, light, oxygen and moisture, as well as having a high evaporation rate, so it is important that they are stored in amber (or dark) glass bottles equipped with tight-fitting tops and, if possible, flow restrictors to avoid accidental spillage. Always be sure to replace the top immediately after use. Never keep essential oils in plastic containers; because they are highly concentrated they can penetrate the plastic and become contaminated.

Oils should be kept at room temperature, which should optimally be about 16 °C (60 °F). The expensive oils, like Neroli, Rose, Jasmine and the citrus oils can be kept in the refrigerator, but they should be at room temperature when being used, so it will be necessary to take them out of the refrigerator in time to allow them to warm up naturally. (Do not attempt to speed up this warming process by placing the bottle in hot water, as this speeds up the oxidation process unnecessarily.) Rose Otto needs special attention since it can be solid at 16 °C. You can help warm it up by rubbing the bottle between your hands. A number of other essential oils have a rather thick consistency and need to be warmed in the same way before use. These oils include Benzoin Resinoid, Cedarwood, Myrrh, Patchouli and Sandalwood. This warming process also enhances the oils' fragrance.

Although a good quality essential oil can last a number of years, most of them reach a point when they start to lose their odour and therapeutic value. The active life-span will vary from oil to oil, and indeed some oils, such as Patchouli, actually get better with age. A general rule is that citrus oils can be kept for up to two years, essential oils from flowers and herbs for between two and four years, and wood oils almost indefinitely. Once essential oils have been blended with carrier oils, however, their shelf life is greatly reduced. It is for this reason that a blend should only be made up in small quantities and used within a few months.

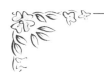

AROMATHERAPY TREATMENTS

Aromatherapy works on the nervous system, helping to promote relaxation and enhance moods. Combined with massage, aromatherapy is a wonderful way to relieve stress, which is often the root cause of many contemporary illnesses. The benefits of aromatherapy can also be derived in a number of different ways, many of which you can use easily at home. An aromatherapist will use massage in a very specific way to treat your particular condition, but in this chapter you will be introduced to the basic massage strokes as a way of combating tension and improving blood circulation. Most of the strokes you will learn can be used on yourself, but for some you will need a partner.

Not only can essential oils help to cure certain conditions, but they can also be used as a preventative measure. The stiffness and pain that often occurs as a result of strenuous physical exercise, such as running, can be alleviated and sometimes eliminated with a massage using an essential oil blend beforehand. A qualified aromatherapist can make up just the right blend for your individual needs.

The role of the professional aromatherapist is to assess the client's situation quickly and decide on a course of treatment, beginning with the aromatherapy massage, and followed by advice on how the client can continue the healing with oils at home. This is what you might experience at the hands of a qualified aromatherapist.

VISITING AN AROMATHERAPIST

A qualified aromatherapist will have undergone a substantial period of training and should be a member of the International Federation of Aromatherapists (IFA). There is a Natural Health Centre in or near most major cities and they are good places to start if you do not already know of a local qualified aromatherapist. If you do not have a Natural Health Centre near you, you can always call the IFA (see Useful Addresses section) and ask them to recommend someone in your area. There are a number of different schools of aromatherapy available, each giving their own diplomas, some requiring less training than others, so it is important that you ensure that the person you choose is properly qualified.

In order for any therapy to work, it is important that you feel comfortable with the therapist. It is the therapist's job to make you feel at ease and convince you that she knows what she is doing.

Remember that you do not have to be ill to visit an aromatherapist! An aromatherapy treatment is a wonderful way of relieving tension and stress in the body which so easily builds up as a result of our busy lifestyles. In addition, an aromatherapy treatment will aid general circulation, increasing the effectiveness of the body to rid itself of toxins.

On the first visit your aromatherapist will want to get to know you by preparing a case history based on a series of questions. These questions will touch upon medical, social, personal and family history. The answers to these questions will help the aromatherapist to evaluate what oils to use as well as those to suggest for home use. A conscientious therapist will refer you to a GP or specialist for problems that may have need of further medical evaluation. The recording of this information is a standard IFA requirement.

Aromatherapy is designed to treat the whole person and so the questions asked should help to determine any physical, mental or emotional tensions. A body assessment is also carried out to determine a number of things including tension areas, skin type, texture and sensitivity. Your aromatherapist will be qualified in body massage, anatomy and physiology. A visual and tactile assessment of the back, face and abdomen combined with a few questions can be of great assistance to the aromatherapist in preparing just the right blend for your own special needs. Of course, a very important aspect is that you actually *like* the smell of the blend which will be used on your body, and so you have the final say. If for some reason you are not pleased with the fragrance, the blend will be adjusted to your liking.

It is important to let the therapist know what you will be doing after your treatment. There are certain oils which have sedative qualities and can dull the senses, so they would be inappropriate to use if you were driving or needed to be particularly alert afterwards.

Remember that the treatment you receive

will be individually designed for you. Your aromatherapist will be happy to discuss any aspect of the session that you may be unsure of, so do not hesitate to communicate your feelings to her, whatever they may be.

It is best not to wash off the oils after your massage, and your therapist should advise you to refrain from taking a bath or shower for at least 6–8 hours. This will allow enough time for full absorption of the essential oils.

For follow-on visits, your aromatherapist will have your chart to refer to and update, thereby keeping an on-going record. Oils used at each treatment may well vary, as they are determined by your current situation.

Although you will need to undress for the treatment (except for underpants), the aromatherapist will ensure that you are kept warm. In fact you will be covered at all times except for the particular part of the body which is being worked on. Your aromatherapy massage will be a total treatment from head to toe. The only thing for you to do is relax and enjoy. After your session, your aromatherapist will give you some time to relax quietly on your own before getting up.

At the end of your session your aromatherapist can provide instructions and guidance for home use of essential oils for your particular needs. You may want to have some of the oils that were used during your treatment, particularly if you found them beneficial (they allowed you to relax, etc.). You should be able to achieve the same atmosphere by using them in your bath or home massage.

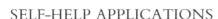

SELF-HELP APPLICATIONS

The rest of this chapter is devoted to describing the various ways to use essential oils. It has been divided into five sections – Massage, Beauty Treatments, Health Treatments, Bathing Treatments and Room Fragrancers. Guidelines are given here regarding the benefits of each method of application and the situations in which you may choose to use it, but in order to discover the most suitable method of treatment and the relevant oils for a particular situation refer to chapters four, five, and six where more specific details are given.

You may find that a range of oils are relevant to your treatment, however, you should never use more than three together in any one blend. Before making your choice of oils it is a good idea to refer to the relevant entries in chapters two and seven for guidance. It is also worth bearing in mind that the body will adjust to the components of an oil and its effect will diminish over time. Varying the oils every two or three weeks will lessen the chance of developing such a tolerance. Above all it is vital that the fragrance of the oil or blend of oils you choose is pleasing to you.

Before you begin to blend your oils and prepare the treatments described on the following pages, you will need to know that there are 20 drops of essential oil in 1 millilitre (ml), and that 1 teaspoon (of the kind used for measuring in cookery) is equal to 5 ml. It will also help you to read pages 65–7 before you decide on the best carrier oil in which to blend your essential oils.

Massage

Massage is one of the oldest forms of treatment; the word itself is French and comes from the Greek 'masseir' meaning 'to knead'. There are many different systems of massage, but the basic principle is to stimulate all of the organs of the body, as well as the circulation of the blood and lymph, thereby helping to clear toxic build up and blockages in the body.

Having an occasional aromatic body massage is a wonderful experience and can leave you feeling great for many days after. For those in-between times there are a number of techniques for relaxation you can use on yourself (such as facial or foot massage), or better still with a partner so that you can take turns working on each other, enjoying the giving as well as the receiving.

There are a variety of basic massage strokes set out on pages 52–6 that you can easily learn and effectively employ to help get rid of tension, particularly in the neck and back regions, alleviate stress and stimulate the circulation. For these you will need a partner.

Both the masseur and the recipient of the massage should remove all jewellery. And if the recipient of the massage wears contact lenses, they also should be removed.

CAUTIONS

Do not massage:
- if any sort of infection or fracture is present;
- over varicose veins or recent scar tissue;
- over bruised or broken skin;
- during pregnancy;
- during or just before menstruation.

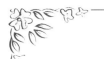

MASSAGE BLENDS

Genuine essential oils are highly concentrated and should not be applied directly to the skin. (See list of oils to be used in small dosages on page 46.) A high-quality vegetable-based carrier oil (see pages 65–7) should be used as a base. Up to 20 drops of one or more essential oils can be added to a 50 ml (1½ fl oz) bottle of carrier oil, i.e. 4 drops per 10 ml. As an average of 4 teaspoons of a massage blend is usually enough to massage a whole body, only a very little is needed to massage a local area. A blend of 10 ml of grapeseed oil with 4 drops of Lavender essential oil is all you need for the massage techniques described here. The different carrier oils available and their properties are discussed on pages 65–7.

Do not forget to use the massage blend on the soles of the feet. This is an excellent way to receive the benefits of the essential oils throughout the body as they are quickly absorbed through the feet, stimulating or relaxing (depending on the oils used) all the corresponding reflex points.

Basic Massage Strokes

The long stroke is a soothing movement useful for applying an essential oil blend. Place a small amount of the oil in the palm of your hand and rub them together so that the oil is spread in both hands. More oil can be added during the massage as required.

This stroke both warms and relaxes the area being massaged and can be repeated several times. It is also a nice way to end a massage.

1 Using the palm and fingers of both hands gently glide over the back starting at the base of the spine and coming up the centre of the back to the neck.

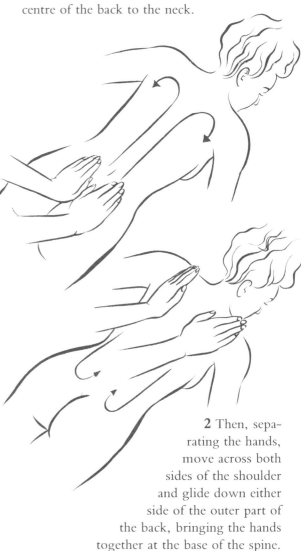

2 Then, separating the hands, move across both sides of the shoulder and glide down either side of the outer part of the back, bringing the hands together at the base of the spine.

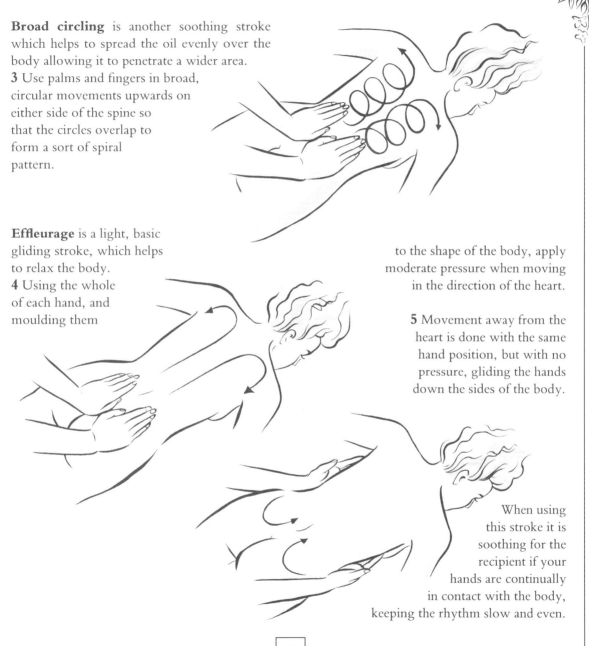

Broad circling is another soothing stroke which helps to spread the oil evenly over the body allowing it to penetrate a wider area.
3 Use palms and fingers in broad, circular movements upwards on either side of the spine so that the circles overlap to form a sort of spiral pattern.

Effleurage is a light, basic gliding stroke, which helps to relax the body.
4 Using the whole of each hand, and moulding them to the shape of the body, apply moderate pressure when moving in the direction of the heart.

5 Movement away from the heart is done with the same hand position, but with no pressure, gliding the hands down the sides of the body.

When using this stroke it is soothing for the recipient if your hands are continually in contact with the body, keeping the rhythm slow and even.

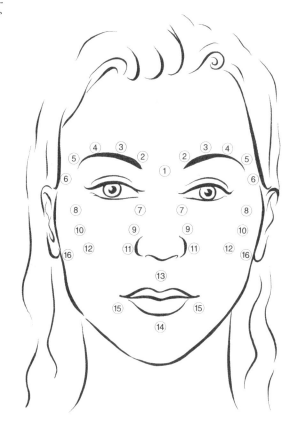

Face Massage

Nothing is more relaxing than a facial massage, especially if it is given by another person. The following steps, however, can be used as a self-help massage technique.

Before you begin massaging ensure that all make-up is removed. First steam the face over a bowl of boiling water for several minutes (covering the head with a towel) then pat the face with a cool moist flannel.

When giving someone else a massage, always start by applying slight pressure and ask for feedback. You can always adjust the pressure accordingly. With your partner lying down start by gently massaging the forehead with your finger tips from the centre working out. End the massage with a soothing facial mask (see page 58).

Left. Apply pressure to each of these points as directed below to give a therapeutic massage.

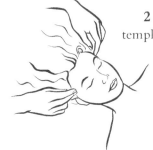

1 Starting from ①, apply gentle pressure with one or two fingers. Then, working across each eyebrow simultaneously, apply quick but smooth amounts of pressure on ②–⑤ with your index fingers.

2 When you reach the temples ⑥ apply pressure for a longer period of time (about 5 seconds). You might want to use two fingers on each side for this.

3 Beginning from ⑦, close to the nose, apply gentle pressure to each point up to ⑫ in turn. Use one finger on each side simultaneously.

4 Place an index finger between the nose and the upper lip ⑬, so that it is parallel to the upper lip, and apply gentle pressure.

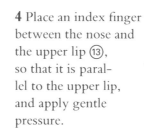

5 Using the same finger, apply pressure to ⑭ below the lower lip and then to points ⑮ in the groove of the chin using both index fingers.

6 Move the fingers up slightly to points ⑯, in line with the lower edge of the ear, applying a small amount of pressure again.

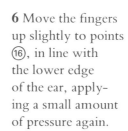

7 Starting from the central point ①, and moving out following the contours of the face, gently run the finger tips across the forehead, then across the eyebrows.

8 Next, starting on either side of the nose run the finger tips very gently under the eyes.

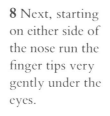
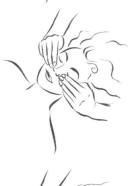

9 Then, from a starting point under the nose ⑬, slowly run the finger tips across the cheeks.

10 Finally, beginning under the mouth at point ⑭, run the finger tips under the mouth and across the chin.

Foot Massage

A gentle foot massage can be both relaxing and stimulating whether given by a partner, or as a therapeutic self-help massage. For maximum benefit, it is best to complete the whole routine on one foot at a time.

1 Holding the foot in both hands, apply a gentle kneading action with the thumbs to the arch on the underside of the foot.

2 Massage the sides of the heel using gentle pressure in a circular movement with the thumb on one side of the heel and the fingers on the other. This can be a very sensitive area for some people, so adjust the pressure accordingly.

3 Holding the foot in one hand, run the thumb of the other along the top of the foot, starting from the big toe and moving up to the ankle. Repeat this from the root of (and between) each toe using moderate pressure.

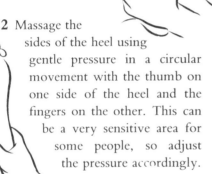

4 Massage both the sole and the sides of the foot with the thumbs and fingers. Moderate pressure is advised, but it can be increased or decreased depending on what the recipient finds comfortable.

5 Holding the foot in one hand, gently squeeze each toe between the thumb and index finger. Starting at the base of the toe draw the fingers towards the top until they join.

6 To finish, caress the foot between both hands with your fingers pointing towards the leg. Slowly and gently pull your hands towards you until they come together off the toes. If you are giving a self-massage end by holding the foot in your hands for a couple of seconds and relax.

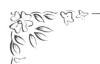

Beauty Treatments

The frenzied pace of life that is characteristic of modern society can play havoc with our skin and hair. Aromatherapy can work in two ways to help improve a lustreless appearance. Firstly, the physical properties of essential oils used in creams, facials and toners can help to correct imbalances in the skin, such as excessive dryness or oiliness, acne, psoriasis and other imperfections or blemishes. And, secondly, the psychological powers of aromatherapy can help to ease tension and combat stress, which is often the root cause of minor skin disorders.

CREAM

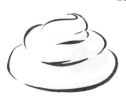

The first known facial cream was created in AD 150 by Galen, a Greek physician. It was a combination of melted beeswax and olive oil with added rosewater. It was called 'cold cream' because it gave a cooling sensation when applied to the skin. Over the years olive oil was replaced with other oils such as almond oil. However, the concept of mixing oil and water is the basic principle of cleansing cream and moisturizing formulas. It seems that oil mixed with water is more helpful in preventing moisture loss than oil alone. Unfortunately, a number of other changes have been made to most of the 'off the shelf' cleansers. To reduce production costs, mineral oil is often used in place of the more expensive vegetable oils. Beeswax is bleached or has dye added to change its natural yellow colour. And, of course, the fragrance from most of these cleansers is produced by synthetic chemicals. All of this detracts from the natural qualities while increasing the cost unnecessarily.

Natural creams can easily be made to suit your personal needs. It is best to make them up in small amounts to ensure their freshness. (Remember that when you mix essential oils with carrier oil their healing properties dissipate after approximately three months.) As there are so many oils that can be used it is best to vary the recipe slightly from batch to batch. Remember also to store creams in air-tight containers, preferably in a cool place.

You can easily make your own cleansing and moisturizing creams by using 20 ml (4 teaspoons) almond oil (you may want to use 5 ml avocado oil and 15 ml almond oil in a moisturizer for added nourishment), 2 tablespoons of grated beeswax, 20 ml distilled or spring water and 8 drops essential oil. The proportion of oil to beeswax can be varied to alter the viscosity of the cream as required.

Recommended essential oils based on skin type

Dry skin: Geranium, Jasmine, Sandalwood
Normal skin: Geranium, Lavender, Jasmine
Oily skin: Bergamot FCF, Cypress, Geranium
Sensitive skin: Chamomile, Neroli, Rose

To make your own cream: shred the beeswax before weighing. Combine this with the almond oil in a pyrex, or heatproof glass bowl and place it in a pan of water over a low heat. Stir the mixture until the beeswax has melted. Remove from the heat and add the water and essential oil. You can use a single essential oil or a combination of two or three oils as long as you do not exceed the recommended number of drops. Whisk vigorously until the mixture becomes creamy then pour immediately into a sterilized jar with a tight-fitting lid. The cream can be kept for about a month without refrigeration.

FACIAL

Effective for all skin types, facial masks are especially beneficial for oily skin as they can deep-cleanse, removing impurities from the skin while replenishing the natural oils and moisture. A good base to use is a mixture of very fine oatmeal and natural yoghurt. The oatmeal is very effective for removing dirt and leaving the skin soft, while the acid in yoghurt is good for killing harmful bacteria. A few drops of an essential oil or a blend of oils chosen according to skin type (see below for some suggestions) are added to the oatmeal–yoghurt mix and blended thoroughly. Using about 2 tablespoons each of yoghurt and oatmeal will make enough for at least two applications. The mixture can be kept covered in the refrigerator for up to one week.

Prior to using a facial mask, especially for oily skin, it may help to steam the face; this will unclog pores in preparation for the deep-cleansing effect of the mask. Fill a deep bowl with boiling water and lean your face over the bowl placing a towel over your head to cover the bowl too. The steam will then penetrate the skin opening pores and bringing any dirt to the surface. For dry skin, a few drops of jojoba or evening primrose oil (see pages 65–6) may be added to help soften the skin.

Apply the mask with your fingers to all the exposed parts of the head. Do not use on or near the eyes. The mask should be left on for about 30 minutes during which time it will dry and harden slightly. It can then be washed off using warm water and a flannel or wash cloth. A splash of cold water or rosewater can be applied to close the pores.

For a coarser consistency suitable for a facial scrub, use oatflakes and $\frac{1}{2}$ teaspoon of bran instead of fine oatmeal. The bran is helpful in removing dirt, grease and dead skin cells as it penetrates the pores. Honey can also be added to the facial mask especially for dry skin, to help soften and nourish the skin.

Recommended essential oils based on skin type

Normal/Dry skin: Chamomile, Geranium, Sandalwood
Oily skin: Cedarwood, Bergamot FCF, Geranium
Mature skin: Frankincense, Myrrh, Sandalwood

TONER

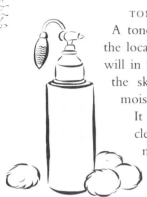

A toner is used to stimulate the local blood supply, which will in turn bring moisture to the skin. It also acts as a moisturizer in its own right.

It is often used after cleansing the skin to remove the last traces of residue such as dead skin cells, grime and make-up. The simplest toner is a splash of cold water to the face, which always has such a fresh, awakening feeling, particularly early in the morning. The only thing lacking is fragrance.

A simple and effective toner can be made from either spring water or distilled water and a few drops of essential oil. Lavender or Rose are excellent choices as both are beneficial to most skin types. Alternatively, you can choose one of the oils listed below, recommended according to skin type. Kept in an atomizer and stored in a cool place, such a toner is a wonderful 'pick me up'.

Recommended essential oils based on skin type

Oily skin: Bergamot FCF, Lavender
Normal/Dry skin: Geranium, Lavender, Roman Chamomile, Rose
Sensitive skin: German Chamomile

To make your own toner: place up to 10 drops (in total) of one or two of the recommended essential oils in 50 ml (1½ fl oz) of spring water, or 2 drops to every 10 ml (⅓ fl oz) of spring water. This blend can be put in an atomizer and sprayed on the skin during the course of the day for a quick, refreshing lift. Be sure to avoid the eye area when applying. It is best to make up the toner in small amounts as it should not be kept for more than three days.

It is advisable not to use regular tap water when making a toner as it generally contains a lot of added chemicals.

HAIR RINSE

Several drops of an essential oil, or blend of essential oils, can be added to 1 litre (2 pt) of warm water and used as a final rinse after washing the hair. Be sure that the oil is completely dispersed in the water before pouring it over the hair.

PERFUME

You can blend your own personal fragrance from your favourite essential oils and enjoy the benefits of their therapeutic qualities as well as the delightful scent. The variety of different combinations are endless. So, remember to keep track of which oils you use (including the number of drops of each oil) or you may end up with the blend that is just right for you but you are unable to duplicate it!

Once you have blended together the desired oils, there are several ways in which the blend may be used. Drops can be added to a pot-pourri or placed on a tissue and tucked in with your clothes. If you want to apply the perfume directly to the skin, dilute it first in Jojoba carrier oil (approximately 10 drops of essential oil per 10 ml of Jojoba oil) and use sparingly.

Health Treatments

In our daily lives we suffer many aches, pains and minor ailments that we may be reluctant to treat with pills or medication. In these circumstances aromatherapy can provide a refreshing alternative. Not only will the use of an appropriate oil in a steambath, compress, inhalation or gargle get to work on the ailment immediately, but the pleasant aroma encountered simultaneously can have an uplifting effect, increasing your ability to fight infection.

STEAMBATH AND SAUNA

One of the main purposes of a sauna or steambath is to help eliminate fluids and toxins from the body. This is, of course, promoted by a combination of increased circulation and opening of the pores, which is encouraged by the hot, steamy atmosphere. By placing 4 to 8 drops (in total) of one or more essential oils on a small piece of cotton wool, the odorous molecules will be released and circulated into the air of a steambath.

For the sauna, 2 drops of essential oil per $\frac{1}{2}$ litre (1 pt) can be added to the water prior to throwing it onto the heat source.

Eucalyptus, Pine Needle or Lemon are the traditional choices of oils used for this purpose, although Tea Tree is another good choice.

COMPRESSES

Depending on the circumstance, either cold or warm compresses may be used. Cold compresses are used to relieve pain, particularly as a result of an injury or wound, as well as to reduce swelling or fever. Hot compresses can help improve circulation, open the pores and reduce pain resulting from internal conditions such as cramps, arthritis and gout.

To make a compress, just add several drops of the desired essential oil or oil blend to a large bowl of water: a maximum of 6 drops to 100 ml (3 fl oz) of water is a good guide. A flannel or wash cloth should then be immersed in the water, wrung out and applied to the skin surface. The cloth can be periodically refreshed with the water mixture, as required. For cold compresses it is usually desirable to replenish the cloth often as the body heat will warm it up quickly. To keep a hot compress at the desired temperature, a hot water bottle can be placed over the cloth. In either case a waterproof material can be used to cover the cloth to prevent making the surrounding area damp.

Once again is it recommended that only 1 drop of any oils that are potential skin irritants be used in compresses (see page 46).

INHALATION

Inhalations can be very effective as decon-gestants. For direct inhalation place 4 to 8 drops of an oil or oil blend on a tissue or hand-kerchief as required.

For insomnia, several drops of a sedative essential oil, or a blend of several, can be sprin-kled on the pillow. Oils for this purpose include Lavender, Neroli and Clary Sage.

STEAM INHALATION

Several drops of the desired essential oil or oils can be added to a steaming bowl of water; up to 8 drops to 1 litre (2 pt) of steaming water is a good guideline, however, be sure to check the chart on page 46 for oils that should only be used in small dosages.

Be sure to agitate the water to dis-perse the oil. Cover your head and the bowl with a towel and with your head about 15 cm (10 in) away from the bowl, breathe in the vapours for a few minutes at a time. It is important to remem-ber that steam inhalation should not be used for too long as that can reverse the initial clearing effect, thereby swelling the mucous membranes and congesting the passages. Steam inhalation is not recommended for those suffering from asthma.

Although Peppermint is excellent to use in a steam inhalation for blocked nasal passages or as a skin decongestant, only 1 drop should be added to a large bowl of hot water for this purpose (see page 46 for other low dosage oils).

There are a number of oils that are effective in a steam inhalation to help alleviate the symptoms of colds and flu. When making a selection bear in mind the time of day. It would not be advisable, for example, to use Cajeput before bedtime as its stimulating properties could prevent sleep. However, blending Cajeput with one of the sedative oils, Lavender for example, would be a useful mix for this purpose.

GARGLE

Gargles are effective for sore throats, strength-ening gums and generally as an effective mouthwash. Just add a drop of essential oil to a glass of warm water. Be sure to disperse the oil by agitating the water vigorously.

Bathing Treatments

Bathing has been considered a way of promot-ing health, looks and general well-being since time immemorial. In a bath, essential oils have a tendency to stay on the surface of the water and the aromatic vapours are breathed in allowing the therapeutic properties to work. Other methods of dispersing essential oils in water, such as in the shower or a local wash, allow the therapeutic molecules to be absorbed by the skin and so enter the bloodstream. Foot-baths are also an excellent way of deriving benefit

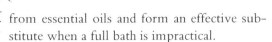

from essential oils and form an effective substitute when a full bath is impractical.

BATH

An aromatic bath is a wonderful way to enjoy the therapeutic properties of essential oils. Between 4 and 6 drops of an essential oil or blend of oils can be added to a full tub of water. Great benefit can be derived from the oil, which penetrates the skin while you are relaxing and breathing in the vapours. Allow at least 10 minutes for complete relaxation. Be sure to disperse the oil before entering the bath.

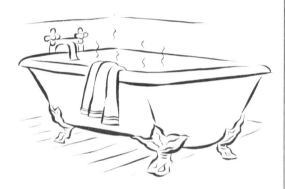

You may prefer to dilute the essential oil before adding it in the bath water, particularly if you have sensitive skin. In this case 4 to 6 drops in total of one or more essential oil can be blended in 1 teaspoon of milk or 2 teaspoons of a quality vegetable or carrier oil (see pages 65–7).

At the onset of a cold, a blend of Orange with any of the spice oils can be very beneficial in a bath. Orange oil contains vitamin C which is stimulating to the immune system, helping it to fight off infection. The spice oils induce perspiration which helps rid the body of toxins. But both Orange and the spice oils can cause skin irritation so use them only in small amounts, diluted in milk or a carrier oil.

Up to four baths a week are recommended as too many can be damaging, drying out the skin and weakening its ability to protect itself from infection.

SHOWER

After cleansing the body, 2 or 3 drops of essential oil may be added to a wet sponge or flannel. This should be briskly rubbed on all or part of your body. You may want to stand under the running water of the shower during this process. If not, be sure you rinse your body

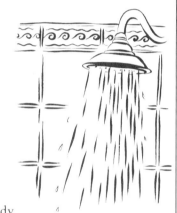

with water afterwards. Any of the flower scents are recommended for this purpose.

FOOT-BATH

This is a wonderful way to relax and refresh tired, sore feet and at the same time stimulate other parts of the body. Reflexology, a form of acupressure applied to the feet, is based on the premise that each organ in the body has corresponding reflex points on the soles of the feet. Although a reflexologist knows how to stimulate each organ individually through the feet, a positive effect can be achieved by simply massaging the whole foot. In addition to stimulating the local blood flow, other parts of the body will more than likely benefit. Alternatively, the feet can be rubbed gently with a loofah while they are in the foot-bath.

For an effective foot-bath add 3 or 4 drops of an essential oil or oil blend to a large bowl of hot water. Make sure that the oil is dispersed before immersing the feet. Allow them to soak for at least 10 minutes. Additional hot water can be added to maintain the temperature, if necessary. Essential oils are quickly absorbed through the feet.

A gentle foot massage, followed by a foot-bath with just 1 drop of Peppermint oil can make feet feel like new after a long hard day. (It is important that **only** 1 drop of this oil is used because of its powerful effect.)

LOCAL WASH

Add several drops of an essential oil or blend of essential oils to a sinkful of warm water. Make sure that the oils are dispersed by agitating the water. A flannel or wash cloth, immersed in the water and gently wrung, can then be applied to the desired area.

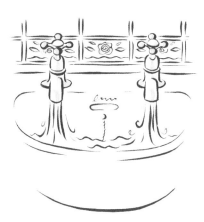

Room Fragrancers

Dispersing essential oil fragrance in the air is a simple, but effective way of experiencing the benefits of aromatherapy. There are a number of ways in which essential oils may be used to disperse fragrance in a room. Here is a selection of the most popular.

VAPORIZER

There are many attractive vaporizers on the market, designed especially for the purpose of evaporating essential oils. They are usually made of ceramic or terracotta, although some glass and bone china ones are also available. They all operate on the same basic principle: a container or small dish holding a water and oil mixture is heated (usually by a nightlight candle although a few designs make use of an electric bulb instead). All you need do is place a few teaspoonfuls of hot water into the vaporizer's dish and add 4 to 6 drops of an essential oil or a blend of oils. Then just light

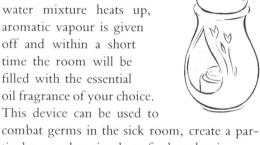

the nightlight or turn on the switch. As the oil and water mixture heats up, aromatic vapour is given off and within a short time the room will be filled with the essential oil fragrance of your choice. This device can be used to combat germs in the sick room, create a particular mood or simply to freshen the air.

FRAGRANCE RING

It is possible to place a drop of oil directly on to a bulb, but in time this may cause the bulb to become sticky and discoloured. There are specially designed fragrance rings available to which water and oil may be added. The ring is placed on a light bulb. If you do use any light bulb method, be sure that the light is switched off and cool prior to adding the ring or oil!

RADIATOR AND HUMIDIFIER

Radiators are another heat source that can be used to disperse fragrance. Several drops of essential oil can be added to a pad of dry cotton wool and placed directly on the radiator. Essential oil drops can also be added to humidifier containers, which disperse moisture in a room.

Alternatively, essential oils can simply be added to a bowl of boiling water and placed in a room. For this method it is best to have all of the windows and doors in the room closed.

ATOMIZER

A plant sprayer or any type of atomizer may also be used to disperse a fragrance into a room. Just place 4 drops of essential oil into 250 ml ($\frac{1}{2}$ pt) of warm water. Pour this mixture into the sprayer, shake and spray. Remember to avoid spraying over wooden furniture.

Many oils are effective for repelling insects. A spray can be made using one or more of any of the following oils (all effective insect repellents): Clove Bud, Eucalyptus, Geranium, Lavender, Lemon, Melissa or Peppermint.

It is important to remember that the olfactory sense adjusts quickly to a scent, so in order to judge the strength of the fragrance in a room it is best to leave the room for a few minutes when the oil is vaporizing and return shortly after.

Many of the oils are effective for reducing, and in some cases actually eliminating, the airborne germs in a room. Although most essential oils have some degree of anti-bacterial or bacteriostatic effect, the most powerful oils to use in a fragrancer for this purpose include Bergamot, Cajeput, Clove Bud, Eucalyptus, Juniper, Lavender, Lemon, Niaouli, Rosemary, Tea Tree and Thyme.

Pine or any of the citrus or flower oils make great air fresheners. They can be used in a vaporizer or as a spray for this purpose.

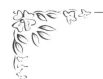

CARRIER OILS

Basically, carrier oils are pure unrefined vegetable oils which complement the use of essential oils in massage and skin care by diluting them so that they can be applied directly onto the skin. Essential oils on their own are too concentrated to use undiluted on the skin with the exception of Lavender oil, which is fully discussed in chapter seven. Vegetable oils used for this purpose should be cold pressed and filtered without the use of solvents. They should also be free of synthetic additives and impurities. Mineral oils should not be used as carrier oils because they do not penetrate the skin and so inhibit the action of essential oils.

THE MAIN CARRIER OILS

Carrier oils facilitate the penetration of essential oils into the body. They are rich in natural fatty acids and can contain a number of vitamins including A and E which help keep the skin supple, regenerated and nourished. The nut oils generally contain potassium and magnesium while sesame seeds are a source of calcium.

SWEET ALMOND OIL

The classic quality carrier oil for massage, Sweet Almond oil has long been valued for this purpose in the East. It is non-irritating and so can be used on sensitive skin types. It gently lubricates and softens the skin and is said to give it elasticity, helping to prevent wrinkling. Contains some B vitamins.

APRICOT KERNEL OIL

This oil helps to maintain healthy skin and surface tissue. Its lightweight quality allows it to penetrate quickly and effectively to soften rough skin. It contains Vitamin A, essential for all skin types.

AVOCADO OIL

This is one of the best penetrating oils and is excellent to use for dry and mature skin types. A large number of vitamins and minerals, including B complex, A and E, makes it a very nourishing oil as well.

To increase the penetration power of Grapeseed or Almond oil, up to 10% of Avocado oil can be included. Avocado oil is beneficial to fatty tissue.

CALENDULA OIL

Calendula oil comes from the Marigold and is infused in a carrier oil, usually Sweet Almond. It contains the essential oil of the plant, which is said to be good for reducing inflammation and renewing body tissue.

COCONUT (LIGHT) OIL

Non-oily in texture this oil makes a good vehicle for most essential oils due to its spreadability. It is more expensive than most of the other general-purpose carrier oils.

EVENING PRIMROSE OIL

Evening Primrose oil is taken from the seeds of the flower and is rich in polyunsaturated fatty acids such as linoleic. It is known for its ability to reduce the rate of blood clotting. It is effective for a number of skin conditions including eczema and psoriasis. A small amount can be included as part of a massage blend or cream for allergic skin problems.

GRAPESEED OIL

This is an exceptionally fine textured oil which allows for easy flow and so it is very good for use as a carrier oil for general massage. As it has virtually no odour of its own, it does not obscure the scent of the essential oils. This makes it a good carrier oil to use with top note essential oils. Its light consistency facilitates the penetration of essential oils into the skin without leaving an oily residue. Grapeseed is also a relatively inexpensive oil to use.

HAZELNUT OIL

A penetrating, nourishing and rich oil which helps prevent skin dehydration.

JOJOBA OIL

A fine penetrating odourless oil which has the consistency of a liquid wax. It is stable and long lasting. It is a good conditioner for all skin types, especially mature skins. Jojoba is also effective for dryness and dandruff and can be massaged on its own into the hair and scalp. The best choice to use as a perfume base because it is the least greasy of the carrier oils.

SESAME OIL

A very light and penetrating massage oil, which is a good source of calcium.

WHEATGERM OIL

Wheatgerm oil is high in Vitamin E, which gives it powerful healing properties. Often included in a blend for its preserving and anti-oxidation properties. For this purpose up to 10% wheatgerm oil may be added to a blend.

Helpful for ageing and dry skin types as well as broken capillaries. It is also an anti-scarring agent and can be used to reduce scar tissue after injury or operations. It can be helpful for facial scarring caused by severe cases of acne. Because of its thick, sticky quality it is best to use blended with either almond or grapeseed oil (25% wheatgerm to 75% almond or grapeseed). Note: There are a number of people who are allergic to wheat, in which case wheatgerm oils should not be used.

BLENDS

Although essential oils have a relatively long life span (several years when kept in proper conditions) when mixed with carrier oils the blend will oxidize much quicker, an important aspect to keep in mind when preparing blends. It is a good idea to make your blends in small amounts and use them within a few months to prevent them from turning rancid. Always store blends in a cool, dark place and preferably in amber bottles.

HOW TO PREPARE A BLEND

For home use, a suitable recommendation would be to add 1 ml (20 drops) of an essential oil or total combination of essential oils (a maximum of three) to 50 ml ($1\frac{1}{2}$ fl oz) of carrier oil (4 drops per 10 ml). Remember that certain essential oils should only be used in low dosages (see chart on page 46). The blend should be inverted several times to ensure that it is well mixed.

It will, of course, be necessary for you to be familiar with the uses of each oil (detailed in chapters two, five, six and seven) in order to make an informed decision as to which essential oil or combination of oils to use. If, for example, you want to have something on hand to use in times of stress, a 5 ml or 10 ml blend of

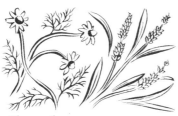

Lavender

Chamomile

equal amounts of Lavender and Chamomile (and for that special touch a few drops of Rose), could be kept available. Whenever you feel the need, up to 6 drops of this blend can be added to a bath. Four drops of the same blend could also be added to 10 ml of one of the carrier oils, Almond or Grapeseed are good choices since they are most often used for massage.

One way of determining which essential oils to use for a blend is to make a list of the various oils that can be used for the condition(s) you want to work on. Be sure to write down alongside each oil their particular note (top, middle or base). Try to make a blend of oils of similar actions belonging to different notes, using, if possible, one from each note. If more than three oils are suitable and you are not sure which to choose, think of the time of day (stimulating for morning, soothing for evening), the emotional situation and especially what the person needs to do afterwards, if the blend is being prepared for a massage.

There are a number of essential oils, such as Cedarwood, Myrrh, Patchouli and Sandalwood which act as fixatives and help delay the evaporation rate of essential oils while keeping the fragrance stable. In fact most of the base notes are suitable for this purpose – a good reason to add a few drops of Rose oil, as it can act as a fixative to your blend.

A good rule of thumb when using essential oils is to start off with low dosages. These can always be increased up to the maximum suggested amount. It is definitely not the case that the more you use the better the effect, in fact it is very often just the opposite!

Along with using the proper oils for the particular situation, it is also important that the smell is pleasing. If you are not happy with the smell of the blend you prepare, it might be a good idea to add a drop of one of the citrus oils. They can add a refreshingly uplifting quality to a heavy blend.

Chapter 4

ESSENTIAL OILS AND BEAUTY CARE

Beauty care means more than using cosmetics to enhance the way you look. It also means taking proper care of the external parts of your body in order to maintain a healthy appearance. The best way to do this is through the use of natural products. Essential oils can have a vital role to play in this process. This chapter sets out the best oils for each skin type plus tips on beauty routines. Various skin conditions, such as eczema and seborrhoea, are discussed and the best treatments recommended. The charts in this chapter have been designed to help you determine which essential oils and method of application best suit the particular condition you wish to affect, whether it is dry skin or lifeless hair. Refer to chapter three for instructions on each method of application. The charts are supported by a wealth of corresponding information, which provides all the detail necessary to make the wisest choices. It is therefore advisable to read the whole chapter before making any decisions.

THE SKIN

The skin reflects the general health of the body and conversely, sensible external care of the skin can play a role in overall health and vitality. It has been suggested that certain essential oils contain natural rejuvenating agents which aid the growth of healthy new cells while helping to eliminate dead ones.

Exposed parts of our bodies are continually subject to external influences; most of these are not very beneficial and in extreme cases are harmful to the skin, particularly in large cities. Because skin is to some extent porous, all kinds of things can penetrate; we not only breathe in atmospheric pollution, for example, it can also enter the body through our skin. The skin can be robbed of vital moisture, too, through exposure to particularly dry environments (centrally heated rooms, for instance) for prolonged periods of time. Climatic conditions also play a part in our skin's health. Sebum is a natural oil produced by the sebaceous glands which provides a thin film of fat over the skin; this slows the evaporation of water and also has an anti-bacterial effect. The production of sebum will normally be greater in natives of hot, dry climates. Extra protection is usually needed when people native to a more moderate climates move to, or even visit, tropical or subtropical habitats.

The use of natural essential oils for skin care can help improve the texture and appearance of the complexion. Ancient

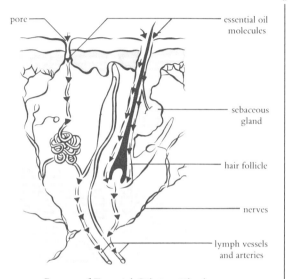

Passage of Essential Oils into Bloodstream

civilizations used them as embalming agents, after all, because of their flesh-preserving properties! In order to obtain the greatest benefit, it is important to ensure that essential oils used for skin care are pure and not synthetically derived (we should be as conscious about what we put on our skin as we ought to be about the nature of the food we eat). Because of the potency of true essential oils, they *should not be applied directly to the skin*, with the exception of Lavender (see page 98–9), but blended with a good quality carrier oil (see pages 65–7). Due to their inherent properties, essential oils penetrate the skin and diffuse into the body via the bloodstream and lymphatic system.

There are a number of oils that have a balancing effect on sebum production and can be used with equal effect on both oily and dry skin. These oils include Geranium and Ylang Ylang. Eczema is a condition that can occur regardless of skin type. There are a number of different causes of this condition, so it is necessary to seek professional assistance in determining its origin. Basically, it is a superficial inflammation of the skin, mainly affecting the epidermis, which causes itching, with a red rash often accompanied by small blisters that weep and become crusted. Scaling, thickening or discoloration of the skin may occur. For the purposes of this book essential oil recommendations for eczema are listed under both dry and oily skin types.

It is important that you read about the various applications of essential oils in chapter three before you attempt to use them. This is particularly important before using any of the essential oils that are marked with a triangle on the charts. The dose used can be of the utmost significance, so be sure to check the cautions listed for the particular essential oils in chapter two as well as the chart on page 46. Melissa, for example, is a valuable oil for eczema as well as for other skin problems; however, only small amounts should be used, otherwise it could have the opposite effect, causing skin irritation.

A number of essential oils make good deodorizers. These oils include Bergamot FCF, Cypress, Juniper, Lavender and Neroli. They can be used in the bath or as a local wash for personal hygiene.

The following information gives suggested uses for essential oils based on skin type.

TREATING SKIN CONDITIONS

DRY SKIN

Dry skin is often of a fine and close-grained appearance and can feel tight. Flaking and peeling are very often a problem when the skin is dry. Early development of facial lines is also characteristic of this skin type. The use of moisturizers to rehydrate the skin is essential.

Chilblains can occur in cold weather when there is poor blood circulation; the skin becomes red, itchy and swollen as a result. Blood circulation needs to be stimulated and there are several essential oils that can help. The best form of treatment is massage, though baths can also be effective.

Stress is often associated with eczema, so it can be beneficial to use calming, relaxing oils. Although massage and creams can be helpful, baths may be preferable, as the fatty carrier oils used in blending massage oils can sometimes irritate the condition.

It is best to avoid harsh cleansers and extremes of temperature. Application of a nourishing facial mask once a week can be very beneficial for those with dry skin. See chapter three for instructions on how to make an essential oil facial mask.

OILY SKIN

This skin type is often shiny in appearance. One of the causes is increased hormonal action that stimulates the sebaceous glands into producing excess sebum. The surplus of natural oils (or sebum) often manifests as acne, particularly in puberty when of other hormonal changes are also taking place in the body. Other conditions include enlarged pores, blackheads and blemishes. Poor elimination causing excessive build-up of toxins is often a contributing factor. The use of harsh synthetic cleansers can make matters worse by removing too many of the natural oils, which only results in overstimulation of the sebaceous glands, which then produce more sebum. Excessive secretion of sebum is known as seborrhoea; this condition can be recognized by enlarged sebaceous glands, especially beside the nose and on other areas of the face.

The causes of psoriasis, which occurs in oily skin types, are not fully understood, although stress seems to play a part. It is a chronic skin disease characterized by itchy, scaly red patches which form on various parts of the body. Essential oils having a sedative and calming effect are usually recommended, as reducing stress seems to have a positive, albeit mainly temporary, effect on psoriasis.

If you suffer from oily skin it is best to avoid harsh cleansers and oily moisturizers. Instead a facial scrub or steaming once a week and a deep-cleansing face mask applied once or twice a week can be beneficial. See chapter three for methods of application.

COMBINATION SKIN

Many people, especially those between the ages of twenty and forty, have an oily chin, nose and forehead (sometimes called the T-zone) while the area around the eyes, cheeks and neck tends to be dry. While different creams can be used on the various parts of the skin according to condition, there are a number of oils which have a balancing effect on sebum, making them a good choice for overall use for this skin type. These oils include Geranium, Lavender, Sandalwood and Ylang Ylang.

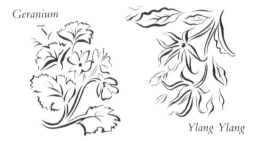

Geranium

Ylang Ylang

A facial scrub on the T-zone and a gentle face mask once or twice a week can be beneficial. Refer to the information on dry and oily skin and choose the appropriate treatment based on the condition of the skin you especially want to treat.

SENSITIVE SKIN

This skin type is very prone to redness and irritation, particularly by chemicals found in the environment as well as complex and artificial skin care products. Sensitive skin is often accompanied by broken capillaries which are usually associated with poor circulation. If you have sensitive skin it is best to stay away from any cosmetics containing alcohol, synthetic chemicals and lanolin.

MATURE SKIN

As a general rule, the skin will be oilier during youth, tending to become drier with age as a result of a decrease in the production of sebum. This reduction in natural oils is one of the conditions responsible for wrinkles. Other characteristics of mature skin include the skin's inability to retain moisture and its loss of elasticity and resilience.

BASIC FACIAL SKIN CARE

It is best to avoid using soap for cleansing the face. Most soaps are very irritating to the skin because they contain synthetically derived chemical fragrances and detergents. In addition, most soaps are too alkaline.

A wax and oil-based cleanser for removing make-up is best. This is because most make-ups are either wax or oil based themselves. A toner can then be used to remove any lingering dirt or grime. A moisturizer protects the skin from extreme temperature variations and loss of moisture, and should be used during the day. All of these products can quite easily be made at home. Of course, essential oils, based on skin type, can be included for added nourishment. Instructions for making your own creams and toners can be found under the appropriate headings in chapter three. You can choose which oil or blend of oils to use based on the charts found on pages 73 and 74, or use one or a blend of the essential oils suggested in chapter three. Although you may want to use different essential oils for moisturizers than for cleansers, the basic formula is the same for both. With the addition of a facial massage and mask treatment (also in chapter three) once or twice a week, you will have everything you need for a healthy glowing skin.

OTHER SKIN CONDITIONS

Skin irritations can stem from a number of situations including stress, use of antibiotics or steroids, food allergies, additives in foods, extreme temperature changes, chemicals, detergents and other synthetic products. It is equally important to determine the cause of the problem as it is to treat the symptoms of any skin condition.

APPLICATION OF ESSENTIAL OIL

SKIN CONDITION	ESSENTIAL OILS TO USE	bath	cold compress	hot compress	cream	room fragrancer	inhalation	local wash	massage	steam inhalation	foot-bath	facial	gargle	perfume
DRY SKIN														
Chapped Skin	Benzoin	●			●				●					
	Myrrh	●			●			●	●					
	Sandalwood	●		●	●			●	●					
Chilblains	Black Pepper ▲								●					
	Cypress	●							●					
	Juniper ▲	●							●					
	Marjoram	●							●					
Dermatitis	Bergamot FCF	●	●		●				●					
	Chamomile	●	●		●				●					
	Geranium	●	●		●				●					
	Lavender	●	●		●				●					
	Neroli	●	●		●				●					
	Rose	●	●		●				●					
Eczema	Bergamot FCF	●	●		●				●					
	Chamomile	●	●		●				●					
	Geranium	●	●		●				●					
	Lavender	●	●		●				●					
	Sandalwood	●	●		●				●					
Tonic	Geranium				●				●					
	Jasmine ▲				●				●					
	Rose				●				●					
	Ylang Ylang				●				●					
OILY SKIN														
Acne	Bergamot FCF	●			●				●					
	Cedarwood	●			●			●	●					
	Juniper ▲	●			●				●					
	Lemon ▲				●			●	●					
	Patchouli				●				●					
	Sandalwood	●			●			●	●					
Seborrhoea	Cypress	●			●				●			●		
	Geranium	●			●				●			●		
	Lavender	●			●				●			●		
	Sandalwood	●			●				●			●		
	Ylang Ylang	●			●				●			●		
Blackheads	Lemon ▲				●			●						
	Peppermint ▲				●			●						
Boils	Bergamot FCF	●		●				●						

Notes ● Indicates the particular application of each oil.
▲ Indicates that oil should be used in small dosages (see page 46).

APPLICATION OF ESSENTIAL OIL

SKIN CONDITION	ESSENTIAL OILS TO USE	bath	cold compress	hot compress	cream	room fragrancer	inhalation	local wash	massage	steam inhalation	foot-bath	facial	gargle	perfume
Boils	Chamomile	●		●				●	●					
	Juniper ▲	●		●				●	●					
	Lavender	●		●				●	●					
Eczema	Bergamot FCF	●	●		●				●					
	Chamomile	●	●		●				●					
	Geranium	●	●		●				●					
	Lavender	●	●		●				●					
	Sandalwood	●	●		●				●					
Psoriasis	Bergamot FCF				●				●					
	Lavender				●				●					
	Sandalwood				●				●					
SENSITIVE SKIN														
	Chamomile	●			●				●					
	Neroli	●			●				●					
	Rose	●			●				●					
MATURE SKIN														
Cell Degeneration	Frankincense				●				●			●		
	Myrrh				●				●			●		
	Neroli				●				●			●		
	Rose				●				●			●		
Dehydration	Chamomile				●				●			●		
	Cypress				●				●			●		
	Geranium				●				●			●		
	Lavender				●				●			●		
	Neroli				●				●			●		
	Sandalwood			●	●				●			●		
Facial Lines	Frankincense				●				●			●		
	Neroli				●				●			●		
Sagging Skin	Patchouli				●							●		
OTHER SKIN CONDITIONS														
Athlete's Foot	Lavender	●			●			●						
	Myrrh	●			●			●						
	Patchouli	●			●			●						
	Tea Tree	●			●			●						
Blisters	Chamomile	●	●					●						
	Lavender	●	●					●						
	Myrrh	●	●					●						
Burns	Chamomile		●					●						

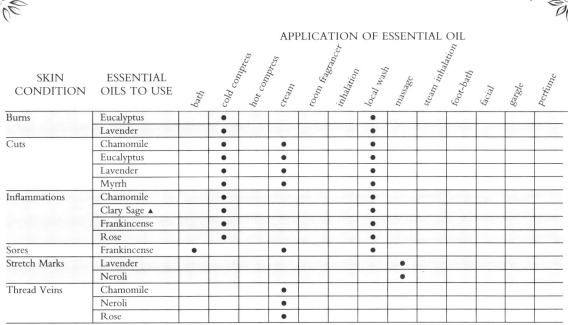

APPLICATION OF ESSENTIAL OIL

SKIN CONDITION	ESSENTIAL OILS TO USE	bath	cold compress	hot compress	cream	room fragrancer	inhalation	local wash	massage	steam inhalation	foot-bath	facial	gargle	perfume
Burns	Eucalyptus		•					•						
	Lavender		•					•						
Cuts	Chamomile		•		•			•						
	Eucalyptus		•		•			•						
	Lavender		•		•			•						
	Myrrh		•		•			•						
Inflammations	Chamomile		•					•						
	Clary Sage ▲		•					•						
	Frankincense		•					•						
	Rose		•					•						
Sores	Frankincense	•			•			•						
Stretch Marks	Lavender								•					
	Neroli								•					
Thread Veins	Chamomile				•									
	Neroli				•									
	Rose				•									

Notes   • Indicates the particular application of each oil.
▲ Indicates that oil should be used in small dosages (see page 46).

THE HAIR

Hair is one of the first things you notice about a person. It is literally the 'crowning glory'. Even though, technically speaking, hair is organically dead material, proper care is essential to keep hair looking healthy. The hair follicles, a sheath of epidermal cells and connective tissue that surround the root of each hair, are very much alive. The hair grows from these follicles on the scalp which need continual nourishment by blood and oxygen. It is important to brush the hair daily to stimulate the blood flow as well as to encourage new hair growth. A natural bristle brush is best and brushing should be done vigorously.

Hair consists of three layers; the outer layer or cuticle is made up of keratin, a protein which protects the hair from bacteria and retains moisture; the cortex which forms the bulk of the hair and contains the pigment which gives the hair its colour; and the medulla, the innermost core, which gives thickness to the hair shaft.

Dry hair can be caused by moisture loss, over-exposure to sun, excessive blow-drying, central heating and chemicals from the application of a number of different processes such as permanent waves and even excessive use of harsh shampoo. This causes the hair to be coarse and brittle, allowing it to be easily damaged. Treatment with Jojoba oil is very nourishing if used once a week before shampooing. Simply pour a small amount into the palm of one hand and, after rubbing both hands together, run both palms and fingers through the hair starting at the scalp. Leave on for about 10–15 minutes. Wash the hair using a non-alkaline shampoo or use the recommended hair rinse for oily hair (see below) after shampooing.

Oily hair is caused by an over-production of sebum. It is necessary to wash hair often because dirt, dust and unpleasant odours from smoking and pollution usually cling to the oil.

After shampooing, a drop of Lemon oil used in the final rinse water can be beneficial to oily hair, as well as helping to ensure that all of the soap is rinsed away. Jojoba oil as a conditioner before the final rinse is equally effective for oily hair as it is for dry.

Dandruff is a common condition in which the scalp is covered with small flakes of dead skin. This is caused by an increase in the normal loss of the outermost layer of skin. Dandruff can occur whether the hair itself is dry or oily. A number of essential oils are useful to help combat dandruff. They include Clary Sage, Patchouli and Rosemary. Rosemary also encourages hair growth.

A hair rinse for dandruff can be very effective. Add 2 tablespoons of apple cider vinegar (preferably organic) and 2 drops of Rosemary oil to 1 litre (2 pt) of lukewarm water. Agitate the water and use as a final rinse after shampooing. Clary Sage is also effective, especially for greasy hair and dandruff, and can be used in place of Rosemary.

Chapter 5

ESSENTIAL OILS AND BODILY HEALTH

Aromatherapy offers a wide range of essential oils with which to help many minor physical disorders, a number of which are listed below. Similar disorders and ways of treating them have been grouped together according to the type of relief that is needed, so pain-relieving treatments, for instance, are grouped under analgesics. Indeed, in most cases, more oils could be added to the list; however, the best choices that can be used safely at home have been indicated. Certain oils should only be used under the direction of an aromatherapist. Please note that the recommended oils are not offered as a cure, but purely as an aid. And, of course, if your condition is serious you should consult a medical practitioner.

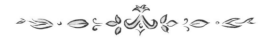

Treating Common Ailments

In this section you will find that many conditions are covered in more than one category. For example, essential oils that are effective for respiratory problems can be found under a number of headings including antiseptics, antispasmodics and expectorants. It is rare that one component of an essential oil can cure a problem. The body is a whole made up of many parts that continually interrelate. Therefore not only do we need to cure the symptom, the outward manifestation of the disorder, but we also need to find the cause and treat it. The root of a disease can be sometimes found in what appears to be a completely unrelated part of the body. But, of course, when you view the body as a whole, then no part can truly be unrelated. In the same way, a plant is made up of many constituents, each contributing to the whole. It follows, then, that the whole plant can work on many different aspects of a problem simultaneously. Lavender oil, for example, is helpful in relieving pain, such as headaches and backache; it also has a calming, sedative quality which helps reduce stress and nervous tension, often the cause of persistent aches and pains. Nature has designed plants to interact with our bodies; by using them in their whole state, as herbs and essential oils, we can help to maintain balance and harmony in our lives.

It is important to read about the properties of each essential oil in chapters two and seven and also how to apply them in chapter three before you attempt to use them. This is vital when using any of the oils that are marked with a triangle, as the dosage can be of the utmost significance. Also be sure to check the cautions indicated in chapters two and seven as well as the chart on page 46.

Where massage is indicated as one of the forms of application, local, topical massage on the affected area is best. As already discused, essential oils should not be used on the skin undiluted. Instead they should be blended with the appropriate carrier oil first (see chapter three).

Remember that when more than one essential oil is recommended for a particular condition using the same application, a blend of up to three oils may be used, rather than choosing just one. Be sure, however, that the dosage is not exceeded for the particular application. To ensure this does not happen and to enable you to use oils with recommended low dosages it is best to first blend a larger quantity of the oils together in a separate bottle. Then use the desired amount, up to the maximum recommended, directly from the blend.

Any definitions provided for various physical conditions and diseases in this chapter and in the glossary are for information purposes only and are in no way meant to be used for self-diagnosis. A reliable diagnosis can only be made by a qualified therapist.

ANALGESIC OILS

Analgesics can be used to relieve a variety of common aches and pains. Essential oils with a warming quality are often used to help reduce pain. These oils generally stimulate circulation, which can in turn help relieve stiffness. Bodily aches and pains can be relieved using essential oils in a foot-bath when it is not convenient to take a full bath.

For headaches, massaging a small amount of the appropriate essential oil (diluted in a carrier oil first) into the temples can be very effective. For migraine it is important to use the essential oils at the first sign, because once a migraine has started, sufferers often cannot stand the smell of essential oils, even their favourites.

The cause of an earache can be very complicated, so it is important to seek proper medical attention. The recommended essential oils indicated on the chart (see page 84) can be used at the first sign of an earache to help alleviate the acute pain. It is important to note, however, that aromatherapy is merely treating the symptom and cannot take the place of medical attention.

Gargling can be effective for a sore throat, using 1 drop of any of the recommended essential oils in a glass of warm water. In the same way a simple mouthwash can be employed to freshen the breath after eating, or while brushing your teeth first thing in the morning. A drop of any of the following oils added to a glass of warm water can be used: Basil, Bergamot FCF, Clary Sage, Fennel, Lavender, Lemon or Orange. Myrrh could be used when bad breath occurs as a result of abnormal gastric fermentations.

ANTI-ALLERGENIC OILS

Essential oils can be used to alleviate the symptoms of allergic reactions. An allergy is a disorder in which the body becomes hypersensitive to particular antigens (toxins) that provoke characteristic symptoms whenever they are subsequently encountered. Different allergies can affect different tissues in the body and may have either local or general effects ranging from asthma and hay fever to severe dermatitis. Antigens can be one of a wide variety of items including dust, pollen and animal hair, as well as certain foods such as wheat, milk or chocolate. The allergy can manifest in a number of ways including catarrh, sudden and recurring colds, watering eyes, constricted air passages, skin irritations, tiredness and mood swings.

Essential oils which are calming and soothing are best to use for allergies as stress is often a factor.

Note: Asthma is sometimes considered to be an allergic condition. Consult the muscular spasm section of the chart on page 86 for recommended oils and their applications. This condition is a serious one and if you suffer from asthma you should seek advice from a qualified practitioner.

ANTI-INFLAMMATORY OILS

Aromatherapy treatment can be an effective way of relieving inflammation. Inflammation of tissue is the body's immediate defensive reaction to infection, injury or physical trauma. It can manifest as pain, heat, redness, swelling and malfunction in the affected area. Blood vessels near the site of the injury will be dilated to increase blood flow locally (so that the white blood cells can engulf bacteria and other foreign particles). Cold compresses usually work best for inflammation due to physical injury, while hot compresses are more suitable for infections and joint inflammations. Massage should not be used as a treatment on inflammations due to injury.

A number of essential oils are beneficial depending on the cause of the inflammation. Generally, Chamomile is the best essential oil for treating inflammations because its azulene content helps to soothe them.

ANTISEPTIC OILS

Antiseptic essential oils can destroy or inhibit the growth of disease-causing bacteria, which lead to infection. They can be used to cleanse wounds in order to prevent infection, and clear infection where it already exists.

ANTI-SPASMODIC OILS

Spasms, or convulsions, are the result of muscular contractions which can be caused by a variety of disorders. Anti-spasmodic oils help to ease or prevent the contractions. Spasms can occur as a result of an upset stomach and nausea. People commonly associate upset stomach with 'something they ate', but that is not always the case. Motion or travel sickness, which results from disturbances of the inner ear, is another cause. Similarly, foul odour, such as greasy food or

smoke from cigars and cigarettes, can quickly induce vomiting once nausea has taken hold.

A pleasant smell can help alleviate or even prevent travel sickness. Prior to embarking on a journey, a blend of Peppermint and Ginger essential oils in a carrier oil can be applied to the stomach and chest. (See chapter three for instructions on how to prepare the blend.) Additionally, just a few drops of one or both of these essential oils can be placed on a tissue and inhaled as necessary during the journey. It is of upmost importance, however, that you find these fragrances pleasing.

Another common cause of nausea is morning sickness. Again, inhaling an appropriate essential oil can often alleviate the feeling.

Spasms can also manifest as respiratory complaints, such as bronchitis. As there are two forms of bronchitis, acute and chronic, it is important to know which you are dealing with before determining the best essential oil and method of application. Acute bronchitis usually occurs as a result of a viral infection of the upper respiratory tract which spreads to the lungs. It usually only lasts for a few days and is characterized by a fever and painful cough. In the early stage, steam inhalation with an appropriate essential oil can be very effective. Elimination of mucus is also important (see 'expectorants', page 82, and also for suggestions regarding chronic bronchitis).

Essential oils associated with relaxation are usually thought to be effective for helping to relieve spasms, but it is important to establish the cause of the spasms first, in order to make the best informed choice. (When selecting oils refer to chapters two and seven to familiarize yourself with any precautions.)

APERITIFS

Aperitifs can be used either to stimulate or depress the appetite. Besides being hungry, a number of factors can stimulate appetite including smell, imagination, anxiety and depression. Conversely, some of these same factors, such as anxiety and depression, can also depress appetite! It really depends on the individual. There may be very deep-seated reasons for an out-of-balance appetite and consultation with a qualified therapist is advised in order to assess the cause. There are certain oils, however, which can help stimulate a sluggish appetite, while others are useful to help temper an overactive one. In some cases the same oil may be used for both situations.

ASTRINGENT OILS

Essential oils can be used to reduce bleeding (or fluid loss) by causing cells to shrink. Although not indicated in the chart (page 87), massage can be used for varicose veins as long as it is above the varicose vein and not directly on or below it. Massage to the surrounding area, not touching the varicose veins, is quite acceptable, but should be done with care. The essential oil can either be blended with a carrier oil or used in a cream.

Diarrhoea can sometimes be caused by fear or stress and for this it would be helpful to use the appropriate essential oils in a bath or mass-

age to help alleviate the situation before it occurs. Prolonged diarrhoea can be dangerous due to the risk of dehydration from prolonged water loss, and it is therefore extremely important that a physician be consulted if it persists for more than two days. Diarrhoea in small children should always be attended to by a qualified doctor.

CARMINATIVE OILS

Carminatives are used to relax the stomach, aiding digestion and curtailing the production of gas. When massaging the abdomenal area with an essential oil and carrier oil blend, always work in a clockwise direction. This is the course that food takes as it is digested.

DETOXIFYING OILS

In addition to using certain essential oils which stimulate circulation, thus helping to rid the body of toxins, daily dry body brushing is also helpful. This is easily done with a loofah or body brush, always stroking towards the heart. Concentrate on the areas of the body characterized by pockets of fatty flab. In this way the lymphatic system is stimulated, encouraging the elimination of toxins from the body.

A common female complaint is cellulite, which is basically the build-up of toxins in the subcutaneous fat giving an 'orange peel' look to the skin. Cellulite is sometimes confused with cellulitis, inflammation of the connective tissue between organs, commonly caused by bacterial infection and usually requiring treatment to prevent it spreading into the blood-

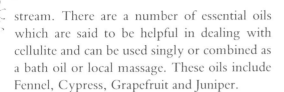

stream. There are a number of essential oils which are said to be helpful in dealing with cellulite and can be used singly or combined as a bath oil or local massage. These oils include Fennel, Cypress, Grapefruit and Juniper.

DIURETICS

Fluid retention is a common complaint, particularly in women; it is treated with a diuretic, which helps eliminate excess fluid and salts from the body. Swollen ankles usually occur after prolonged standing, most often in hot weather. A cold compress of Geranium essential oil is probably the best remedy for this type of fluid retention.

EXPECTORANTS

Expectorants are usually found in cough mixtures. They act by increasing the bronchial secretion or making it less viscous, so helping to remove it from the respiratory system. Some commercial expectorants work by causing irritation to the lining of the stomach which provides a stimulus for the reflex production of sputum by the glandular cells in the bronchial mucous membrane. Essential oils work by ridding the body of excess mucus in a soothing way.

Chronic bronchitis is a long-term condition, characterized by a permanent cough with sputum and breathlessness as a result of exertion. Certain cells are destroyed and replaced by ones that do not have the same protective properties, thus there is a reduced defence against infection. Although part of the ultimate remedy needs to be a close look at diet, proper use of essential oils can be very helpful, particularly those that have a stimulating effect on the immune system in addition to those which help reduce the amount of mucus production. See 'anti-spasmodic oils' for information on acute bronchitis.

EMMENAGOGUES

Certain essential oils, Geranium, for example, seem to have an influence on the secretion of hormones and are therefore, effective to use whether stimulation or balancing of menstruation is required. Clary Sage has been used for painful and scanty periods, post-natal depression as well as to help encourage labour during childbirth (use in a fragrancer for this purpose would be recommended).

There are a number of essential oils that should not be used during the first few months of pregnancy, particularly those that stimulate menstruation such as Clary Sage, Marjoram and Rosemary. If there is any question of possible pregnancy, it is best to consult with a qualified practitioner.

A list of essential oils that can be used for painful periods is also provided, although not all of these oils can be considered to be emmenagogues.

FEBRIFUGE

Increased temperature is one of the defensive mechanisms used by the body to help discard toxins. A number of essential oils help induce sweating, which can assist in this process, and,

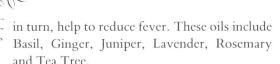

in turn, help to reduce fever. These oils include Basil, Ginger, Juniper, Lavender, Rosemary and Tea Tree.

To keep the body below a dangerous temperature level, one of a number of cooling oils can be used (about 1 drop in a cool bowl of water for a compress). These oils include Eucalyptus, Lavender and Peppermint.

FUNGICIDAL OILS

Certain essential oils can help to fight fungal infections by inhibiting the growth of fungi and yeast. The fungus *Candida albicans*, commonly known as thrush, can affect the mouth as well as the vagina. This condition can flourish after a course of antibiotics because much of the 'friendly flora' in the intestinal tract is destroyed by the antibiotics. It is this 'friendly flora' that keeps *Candida albicans* under control.

GALACTAGOGUES

Breast-feeding mothers may have problems with milk flow and wish to increase it with a galactagogue. Fennel essential oil contains a plant hormone which has a similar action to oestrogen, making it very effective for a number of female conditions including stimulating the flow of milk in nursing mothers.

HYPERTENSIVE OILS

Certain oils act as hypertensives, increasing blood pressure when it has fallen below the normal level. Rosemary works in a normalizing rather than stimulating capacity whereas

Thyme is more stimulating and should only be used under the guidance of a qualified practitioner. A number of other stimulating oils are listed.

HYPOTENSIVE OILS

From time to time we all have a flare up of blood pressure, particularly when we get angry or frustrated and need something to calm ourselves down. A soothing bath with one or a blend of relaxing oils can be just the answer to help lower blood pressure. This can go equally well after a stressful day at work or having to deal with heavy traffic. Massage is another very effective way of reducing tension that can lead to high blood pressure, and a regular massage by a professional aromatherapist is an excellent idea. Continued high blood pressure, on the other hand, causes strain to the blood vessels and heart, making it a problem that should be dealt with by a qualified practitioner.

NERVINES

Calming and relaxing essential oils can have a positive effect on the nervous system and help to relieve tension. Oils that can induce sleep, such as Chamomile, are also a good choice.

TONICS

A tonic can be strengthening for a specific body organ or the whole body in general. Stimulating oils are best suited for this purpose, particularly those which help the immune system. These are useful during convalescence to help restore the body's vitality.

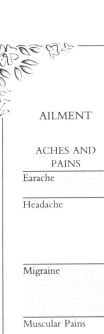

APPLICATION OF ESSENTIAL OIL

AILMENT	ESSENTIAL OILS TO USE	bath	cold compress	hot compress	cream	room fragrancer	inhalation	local wash	massage	steam inhalation	foot-bath	facial	gargle	perfume
ACHES AND PAINS														
Earache	Chamomile			●					●					
	Lavender			●					●					
Headache	Basil ▲					●	●		●					
	Chamomile		●			●	●		●					
	Lavender		●			●	●		●					
	Lemongrass ▲		●						●					
	Peppermint ▲		●						●					
Migraine	Basil ▲					●			●					
	Lavender		●			●			●					
	Rosemary					●			●					
	Peppermint ▲		●			●								
Muscular Pains	Black Pepper ▲								●					
	Lemongrass ▲								●					
	Marjoram								●					
Arthritis	Chamomile	●		●					●					
	Lavender	●		●					●					
	Pine ▲			●					●					
	Rosemary	●		●					●					
Foot Ache	Peppermint ▲										●			
Lower Back Pain	Chamomile	●		●					●					
	Rosemary	●		●					●					
	Lavender	●		●					●					
Rheumatic Pain	Chamomile	●		●					●					
	Eucalyptus	●		●					●					
	Ginger ▲			●					●					
	Lavender	●		●					●					
	Marjoram			●					●					
	Rosemary	●		●					●					
Premenstrual Tension	Bergamot FCF	●		●				●	●					
	Chamomile	●		●				●	●					
	Geranium	●		●				●	●					
	Rose	●		●				●	●					
Sore Throat	Benzoin									●				
	Tea Tree								●	●			●	
	Lavender								●	●			●	
	Lemon ▲												●	
Toothache	Chamomile			●										
	Clove Bud ▲			●										

APPLICATION OF ESSENTIAL OIL

AILMENT	ESSENTIAL OILS TO USE	bath	cold compress	hot compress	cream	room fragrancer	inhalation	local wash	massage	steam inhalation	foot-bath	facial	gargle	perfume
ALLERGIES														
Hay Fever	Chamomile						●		●					
	Eucalyptus						●		●					
	Lavender						●		●					
	Melissa ▲						●		●					
Skin Irritation	Chamomile	●			●									
	Lavender	●			●									
	Melissa ▲	●			●									
INFLAMMATION														
Abscess	Chamomile			●										
	Lavender			●										
	Myrrh			●										
Arthritis	Chamomile	●		●					●					
	Lavender	●		●					●					
Bursitis	Chamomile	●		●					●					
	Lavender	●		●					●					
Inflamed Mucous Membrane	Myrrh	●					●		●					
	Sandalwood			●					●	●				
Inflamed Wounds	Geranium		●											
	Myrrh		●											
Boils	Chamomile			●										
Splinters	Chamomile		●											
	Myrrh		●											
INFECTION														
Aphthae	Geranium												●	
	Myrrh												●	
Catarrh	Frankincense	●		●		●	●		●					
Chest Infection	Jasmine ▲	●		●		●	●		●					
	Myrrh	●		●		●	●		●					
	Pine ▲					●	●			●				
Colds	Cinnamon Leaf ▲	●				●	●							
	Eucalyptus	●					●							
	Orange ▲	●					●				●			
	Peppermint ▲	●					●		●					
	Rosemary	●					●		●					
Nasal Infection	Tea Tree						●			●				

Notes ● Indicates the particular application of each oil.
▲ Indicates that oil should be used in small dosages (see page 46).

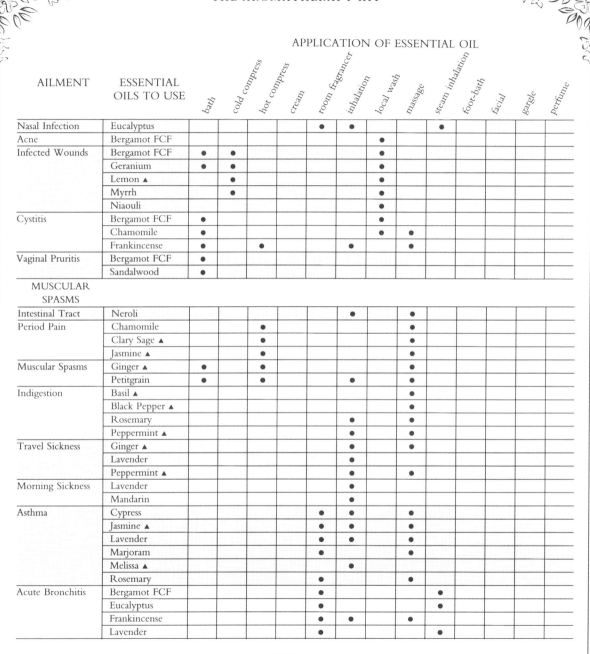

APPLICATION OF ESSENTIAL OIL

AILMENT	ESSENTIAL OILS TO USE	bath	cold compress	hot compress	cream	room fragrancer	inhalation	local wash	massage	steam inhalation	foot-bath	facial	gargle	perfume
Nasal Infection	Eucalyptus					●	●			●				
Acne	Bergamot FCF							●						
Infected Wounds	Bergamot FCF	●	●					●						
	Geranium	●	●					●						
	Lemon ▲		●					●						
	Myrrh		●					●						
	Niaouli							●						
Cystitis	Bergamot FCF	●						●						
	Chamomile	●						●	●					
	Frankincense	●		●			●		●					
Vaginal Pruritis	Bergamot FCF	●												
	Sandalwood	●												
MUSCULAR SPASMS														
Intestinal Tract	Neroli						●		●					
Period Pain	Chamomile			●					●					
	Clary Sage ▲			●					●					
	Jasmine ▲			●					●					
Muscular Spasms	Ginger ▲	●		●					●					
	Petitgrain	●		●			●		●					
Indigestion	Basil ▲								●					
	Black Pepper ▲								●					
	Rosemary						●		●					
	Peppermint ▲						●		●					
Travel Sickness	Ginger ▲						●		●					
	Lavender						●							
	Peppermint ▲						●		●					
Morning Sickness	Lavender						●							
	Mandarin						●							
Asthma	Cypress					●	●		●					
	Jasmine ▲					●	●		●					
	Lavender					●	●		●					
	Marjoram					●			●					
	Melissa ▲						●							
	Rosemary					●			●					
Acute Bronchitis	Bergamot FCF					●				●				
	Eucalyptus					●				●				
	Frankincense					●	●		●					
	Lavender					●				●				

APPLICATION OF ESSENTIAL OIL

AILMENT	ESSENTIAL OILS TO USE	bath	cold compress	hot compress	cream	room fragrancer	inhalation	local wash	massage	steam inhalation	foot-bath	facial	gargle	perfume
Acute Bronchitis	Marjoram			●		●	●		●					
	Rosemary			●		●	●		●	●				
	Sandalwood					●	●		●	●				
Coughs	Cypress			●		●	●		●					
	Eucalyptus			●		●	●		●	●				
	Lavender			●		●	●		●	●				
	Melissa ▲						●							
	Sandalwood			●		●	●		●	●				
Palpitations	Neroli						●		●					
Shortness of Breath	Frankincense						●							
APPETITE DISORDERS														
Lack of Appetite	Bergamot FCF					●	●		●					●
	Chamomile					●	●		●					●
	Fennel ▲					●	●							
	Ginger ▲					●	●							
Excessive Appetite	Bergamot FCF	●				●	●		●					●
	Fennel ▲					●	●							
FLUID LOSS														
Bleeding Gums	Cypress												●	
	Lemon ▲												●	
Diarrhoea	Chamomile	●						●	●					
	Geranium	●						●	●					
	Lavender	●						●	●					
	Neroli	●						●	●					
Haemorrhoids	Cypress	●			●			●						
	Geranium	●			●			●						
	Juniper ▲	●			●			●						
	Myrrh	●			●			●						
Nose Bleeds	Lemon ▲		●											
Varicose Veins	Cypress	●	●											
	Lavender	●	●											
	Juniper ▲	●	●											
DIGESTIVE DISORDERS														
Flatulence	Bergamot FCF	●		●				●	●					
	Chamomile	●		●				●	●					

Notes ● Indicates the particular application of each oil.
▲ Indicates that oil should be used in small dosages (see page 46).

APPLICATION OF ESSENTIAL OIL

AILMENT	ESSENTIAL OILS TO USE	bath	cold compress	hot compress	cream	room fragrancer	inhalation	local wash	massage	steam inhalation	foot-bath	facial	gargle	perfume
Flatulence	Fennel ▲	●		●			●							
	Melissa ▲	●					●		●					
	Nutmeg ▲								●					
	Orange ▲						●		●					
	Rosemary	●							●					
Indigestion	Bergamot FCF	●		●			●		●					
	Chamomile	●		●			●		●					
	Clary Sage ▲	●		●			●		●					
	Fennel ▲	●		●			●							
	Ginger ▲			●					●					
	Marjoram	●		●			●		●					
	Myrrh								●					
	Peppermint ▲	●		●			●		●					
	Petitgrain	●					●		●					
Intestinal Cramps	Marjoram	●					●		●					
BUILD-UP OF TOXINS														
	Cypress	●			●				●					
	Fennel ▲	●			●				●					
	Grapefruit ▲				●				●					
	Juniper ▲	●			●				●					
	Rose	●			●				●					
FLUID RETENTION														
Swelling	Chamomile	●	●						●					
	Cypress	●	●						●					
	Geranium	●	●				●		●					
	Juniper ▲	●	●						●					
	Patchouli	●	●						●					
Urinary Disorders	Eucalyptus	●		●			●		●					
	Fennel ▲	●		●			●							
	Juniper ▲	●		●					●					
RESPIRATORY DISORDERS														
Chronic Bronchitis	Benzoin	●					●		●					
	Myrrh	●					●		●					
	Frankincense	●					●		●					
Congestion/Catarrh	Cedarwood	●				●	●		●					
	Cypress					●	●							

APPLICATION OF ESSENTIAL OIL

AILMENT	ESSENTIAL OILS TO USE	bath	cold compress	hot compress	cream	room fragrancer	inhalation	local wash	massage	steam inhalation	foot-bath	facial	gargle	perfume
Congestion/Catarrh	Eucalyptus	●				●	●		●	●				
	Frankincense					●	●							
	Myrrh	●					●		●					
	Peppermint ▲					●	●			●				
	Pine ▲					●	●			●				
	Sandalwood					●				●				
MENSTRUAL PROBLEMS														
Painful Periods	Chamomile	●		●			●		●					
	Clary Sage ▲	●		●			●		●					
	Marjoram	●		●			●		●					
	Lavender	●		●			●		●					
Scanty Periods	Basil ▲	●							●					
	Juniper ▲	●							●					
	Myrrh	●							●					
	Peppermint ▲	●							●					
	Rose	●							●					
Post-Natal Depression	Clary Sage ▲			●		●	●							
FEVERS														
	Basil ▲					●	●		●					
	Eucalyptus	●	●			●	●		●					
	Ginger ▲	●							●					
	Juniper ▲					●	●		●					
	Lavender	●	●			●	●		●					
	Lemon ▲					●	●		●					
	Orange ▲					●	●		●					
	Peppermint ▲	●	●			●	●		●					
	Rosemary	●				●	●		●					
	Tea Tree	●				●	●		●					
FUNGAL INFECTIONS														
Thrush	Lavender	●						●						
	Myrrh	●						●						
	Tea Tree	●						●						

Notes ● Indicates the particular application of each oil.
▲ Indicates that oil should be used in small dosages (see page 46).

APPLICATION OF ESSENTIAL OIL

AILMENT	ESSENTIAL OILS TO USE	bath	cold compress	hot compress	cream	room fragrancer	inhalation	local wash	massage	steam inhalation	foot-bath	facial	gargle	perfume
BREAST-FEEDING PROBLEMS														
Low Milk Supply	Fennel ▲	●							●					
	Jasmine ▲	●							●					
BLOOD PRESSURE FLUCTUATIONS														
Low Blood Pressure	Black Pepper ▲								●					
	Rosemary	●					●		●					
	Peppermint ▲						●		●					
High Blood Pressure	Chamomile	●				●			●					
	Lavender	●				●			●					
	Marjoram	●				●			●					
	Neroli	●				●			●					
	Rose	●				●			●					
	Ylang Ylang	●							●					
TENSION														
	Chamomile	●				●	●		●					
	Lavender	●				●	●		●					
	Marjoram	●				●	●		●					
	Melissa ▲	●				●	●		●					
	Rosemary	●				●	●		●					
GENERAL DEBILITY														
Low Vitality	Cinnamon Leaf ▲	●					●		●					
	Clary Sage ▲	●				●	●		●					
	Fennel ▲	●					●		●					
	Geranium	●				●	●		●					
	Juniper ▲	●							●					
	Lemongrass ▲	●				●	●		●					
	Melissa ▲	●				●	●		●					
	Petitgrain	●				●	●		●					
	Rose	●				●	●		●					
Kidney Disorders	Cedarwood	●							●					
	Clary Sage ▲	●					●		●					
	Geranium	●				●	●		●					

Notes ● Indicates the particular application of each oil.
▲ Indicates that oil should be used in small dosages (see page 46).

Chapter 6

ESSENTIAL OILS AND THE MIND

The holistic approach to preventative, as well as curative, healing needs to take the mind into consideration in order to be totally successful. Healing needs to occur on both levels – mind and body – to be completely effective. This aspect of healing is very often overlooked by conventional methods. The therapist, orthodox or complementary, can only act as a facilitator, the actual healing is dependent upon the individual. To this end, a knowledge of what we can do for ourselves, when we feel out of balance mentally, can have a tremendous effect on our whole being. Essential oils can have a powerful effect on our mental states, which in turn affects our health and vitality.

BALANCING EMOTIONS

Certain hormones produced in the body can have a balancing effect on emotional situations. The production of these hormones can be stimulated with specific essential oils indicated in the charts on pages 94–5. Lethargy can be relieved by using one, or a blend of several of the stimulating essential oils in a room fragrancer or bath, for example. Similarly, a relaxing bath of one or a blend of the more sedative oils may be just the answer after a busy or stressful day to help you relax and unwind.

The use of essential oils to balance hormones need not be restricted to home use only. There are a number of essential oils that can help clear the mind and indeed enhance memory. A bottle of Rosemary or Basil on your desk, for instance, can be a great asset if you work in an office environment. They can also be useful if kept in the car glove compartment and occasionally sniffed during a long tedious drive. The chart on page 94 outlines a number of emotional and mental conditions with a list of essential oils and methods of application recommended to re-establish the balance.

Once again, it is important that you read about how to apply essential oils in chapter three before you attempt to work with them, especially if you intend to use a bath or massage as the dose used can be of the utmost significance. Particular attention should be paid to oils in the chart marked with a triangle. If used in excess they can cause irritation when in contact with the skin.

STIMULATING AND UPLIFTING OILS

There are a number of oils which can have a stimulating as well as uplifting effect. It is always important that you find the scent pleasing in order to gain benefit from the oil, and so the choice of essential oils will vary from person to person. If, however, depression is a factor, then more thought needs to be given to both the symptoms and the cause in order to choose the right essential oils.

Depression can stem from many sources and manifest in equally as many different ways. Although there are a number of essential oils that are generally uplifting, an assessment of what form the depression is taking is necessary before deciding which oils to choose. If someone is generally lethargic, then an oil which has sedative properties would not be suitable. However, for those where the depression manifests as restlessness, then a sedative oil could be the best choice. It is for this reason that a list of sedative essential oils is included.

CALMING AND SOOTHING OILS

Anxiety is another of the common problems of our modern Western society. It can manifest itself in a number of ways and is very closely related to, and may be indistinguishable from, stress. Creating a relaxing environment is the key to controlling anxiety. Here again, one or a blend of a few of the sedative essential oils can be very helpful for calming nerves and reducing blood pressure.

DE-STRESSING AND RELAXING OILS

Stress features high on the list of most prevalent problems facing Western society. It can be defined as any factor threatening the body's health or having an adverse effect on its functioning. All forms of injury, disease and worry fit into this definition. Constant stress brings about changes in the balance of hormones in the body. Stress relating to one cause can, in turn, lead to other stress problems. For example, constant worry and anxiety (common forms of stress) can lead to a number of physical diseases, depending on the individual's personal weaknesses. One of the ways to cope with stressful situations is to calm the mind by inducing a peaceful and serene atmosphere. The use of certain essential oils can help to create such an environment.

For insomnia, a few drops of one of the recommended essential oils placed on the pillow can be very soothing and help induce sleep. Clary Sage has powerful sedative qualities; however, it should never be used in association with alcohol, particularly for insomnia as it can cause nightmares.

MIND CLARIFYING OILS

There are reports that when used prior to bedtime Clary Sage can induce dramatic and colourful dreams and even help promote lucid dreaming. (Lucid dreaming is a remarkable mental state in which one becomes fully conscious within a dream, but without waking up. Considerable research is being conducted on this potentially important state of mind.) Several drops can be placed on the pillow to inhale or it can be used in a fragrancer, which can be set up about 20 minutes before going to bed so that the scent permeates the room.

Essential oils can also be used in a fragrancer or as an inhalation to enhance or correct other mental processes. Both Basil and Peppermint, for example, are useful for clarifying the mind and stimulating concentration. Ginger and Rosemary are also known mind clarifiers and memory enhancers. Clove Bud is another oil used to treat poor memory. Frankincense has long been used as an aid for meditation, by permeating the room with its aroma.

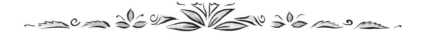

APPLICATION OF ESSENTIAL OIL

MENTAL STATE	ESSENTIAL OILS TO USE	bath	cold compress	hot compress	cream	room fragrancer	inhalation	local wash	massage	steam inhalation	foot-bath	facial	gargle	perfume
DEPRESSION														
Melancholy	Basil ▲					●	●		●					
	Jasmine ▲	●				●	●		●					●
Lethargy	Eucalyptus	●				●	●		●					
	Juniper ▲	●				●	●		●					
	Lemongrass ▲	●				●	●		●					
	Orange ▲	●				●	●		●					
	Peppermint ▲	●				●	●		●					
	Rosemary	●				●	●		●					
Restlessness	Bergamot FCF	●				●	●		●					
	Chamomile	●				●	●		●					
	Clary Sage ▲	●				●	●		●					
	Jasmine ▲	●				●	●		●					
	Lavender	●				●	●		●					
	Marjoram	●				●	●		●					
	Neroli	●				●	●		●					
	Rose	●				●	●		●					
	Sandalwood	●				●	●		●					
	Ylang Ylang	●				●	●		●					
Inertia	Cinnamon Leaf ▲	●				●	●		●					
	Ginger ▲	●				●	●		●					
ANXIETY														
Nervousness	Cypress	●				●	●		●					
	Lavender	●				●	●		●					
	Neroli	●				●	●		●					
	Sandalwood	●				●	●		●					
High Blood Pressure	Chamomile	●				●	●		●					
	Lavender	●				●	●		●					
	Neroli	●				●	●		●					
	Marjoram	●				●	●		●					
	Rose	●				●	●		●					
	Ylang Ylang	●				●	●		●					
Irritability	Bergamot FCF	●				●	●		●					
	Chamomile	●				●	●		●					
	Clary Sage ▲	●				●	●		●					
	Jasmine ▲	●				●	●		●					
	Lavender	●				●	●		●					
	Marjoram	●				●	●		●					
	Neroli	●				●	●		●					
	Rose	●				●	●		●					

APPLICATION OF ESSENTIAL OIL

MENTAL STATE	ESSENTIAL OILS TO USE	bath	cold compress	hot compress	cream	room fragrancer	inhalation	local wash	massage	steam inhalation	foot-bath	facial	gargle	perfume
Irritability	Sandalwood	●				●	●		●					
	Ylang Ylang	●				●	●		●					
Tension	Benzoin					●	●		●					
	Cedarwood	●				●	●		●					
	Geranium	●				●	●		●					
	Lavender	●				●	●		●					
	Melissa ▲					●	●		●					
	Petitgrain	●				●	●		●					
	Ylang Ylang	●				●	●		●					
STRESS														
Nervous Tension	Bergamot FCF	●				●	●		●					
	Benzoin					●	●		●					
	Chamomile	●				●	●		●					
	Lavender	●				●	●		●					
	Marjoram	●				●	●		●					
	Neroli	●				●	●		●					
	Sandalwood	●				●	●		●					
Hormonal Imbalance	Chamomile	●				●	●		●					
	Geranium	●				●	●		●					
	Lavender	●				●	●		●					
	Rose	●				●	●		●					
Insomnia	Chamomile	●				●	●		●					
	Clary Sage ▲	●				●	●		●					
	Lavender	●				●	●		●					
	Marjoram	●				●	●		●					
	Neroli	●				●	●		●					
	Sandalwood	●				●	●		●					
	Ylang Ylang	●				●	●		●					
Agitation	Bergamot FCF	●				●	●		●					
	Chamomile	●				●	●		●					
	Clary Sage ▲	●				●	●		●					
	Jasmine ▲	●				●	●		●					
	Lavender	●				●	●		●					
	Marjoram	●				●	●		●					
	Neroli	●				●	●		●					
	Rose	●				●	●		●					
	Sandalwood	●				●	●		●					

Notes ● Indicates the particular application of each oil.
▲ Indicates that oil should be used in small dosages (see page 46).

Chapter 7

YOUR AROMATHERAPY KIT

The collection of oils in this kit have been especially chosen to provide an introduction to the home use of essential oils. They offer a wide range of applications to help numerous common ailments, skin conditions and mental disorders. This chapter presents detailed information on each of the essential oils in the kit, plus recipes and suggested applications to aid a variety of everyday complaints. In many cases more than one essential oil may be appropriate, in which case you may either choose to use one particular oil, or a blend of the relevant oils. You can use equal amounts of the recommended oils for the blend, or more of one than another to match your preferred fragrance, unless otherwise instructed. All methods of application suggested here are fully described in chapter three.

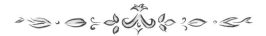

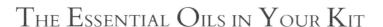

THE ESSENTIAL OILS IN YOUR KIT

There are five 2.5 ml bottles of essential oil in your *Aromatherapy Kit*: Eucalyptus, Geranium, Lavender, Rosemary and Tea Tree. Each bottle is fitted with a flow-restrictor to guard against accidental spillage and control the amount of oil dispensed. The following information reveals the diverse nature of their applications.

EUCALYPTUS *Eucalyptus globulus*
Top note; distilled from the leaves

ORIGINS

One of the tallest trees known, with well over 500 species, the Eucalyptus is native to Australia and Tasmania where it is also known as the Blue Gum Tree, as well as the Fever Tree because of its antiseptic qualities. The name *Eucalyptus* derives from the Greek 'eucalyptos' which means 'a well and a lid'; the sepals and petals fuse together forming a cap resembling a well with a lid. This 'lid' literally gets thrown off when the flower expands. *Globulus* means 'little globe' and refers to the shape of the fruit. The leaves, which are leathery in texture, are studded with glands which contain the fragrant volatile oil. The aborigines traditionally used the leaves to bind wounds. The tree was made known to Europe in the mid-nineteenth century by Baron Ferdinand von Muller, a German botanist who was a director of the Botanical Gardens in Melbourne, Australia (1857–73). It has since been cultivated in many subtropical climates including Egypt, Spain, China and India. Von Muller suggested that the oil resembled Cajeput oil and could be used as a disinfectant. It was also discovered that the roots of the Eucalyptus had a very strong drying effect on the soil. This finding was made as a result of some seeds being planted in a rather marshy district of Algiers. About five years after the seeds had been planted the surrounding area was dry. Eucalyptus has been planted in swampy areas, which attract malaria-bearing mosquitoes, because of its ability to absorb large quantities of water from the soil. In the last century the tree has become established as a source of timber, shade and soil drainage in addition to the essential oil it provides.

MAIN CONSTITUENTS

Aldehyde: citronellal; ketone: cineole (or eucalyptol); terpenes: aromadendrene, camphene, fenchene, phellandrene, pinene.

QUALITIES

One of the best antiseptic oils and anti-viral agents. Best known for its effect on colds and catarrh. Excellent for aches and pains. A stimulating oil.

TRADITIONAL USES

Used for colds, fevers, snake bites, rheumatism and muscular pains. Traditionally used as a general healer by aborigines. Frequently used in saunas to cleanse the atmosphere. Popular ingredient in the pharmaceutical industry for inhalants which are marketed to relieve congestion, catarrhal colds as well as chronic bronchitis.

CAUTIONS

Should be used sparingly as it could irritate the skin if used in high dosages. Avoid if using homoeopathic remedies.

GERANIUM *Pelargonium graveolens*
Middle note; distilled from the leaves

ORIGINS

Geranium comes from the Greek word 'geranos', for 'crane'. Indeed, it was known as Cranesbill in America. Native to The Cape of Good Hope, South Africa, it is cultivated widely in countries including Italy, China, Egypt, Spain, France, Morocco, Réunion and Japan. It is also known as Rose Geranium, because its fragrance is reminiscent of roses, and is sometimes used as a substitute for the more expensive Rose oil. The oil was introduced to Britain from Cape Province in 1632. Its potential in perfumery was recognized in France in the mid-nineteenth century. It was believed that Geranium kept away evil spirits.

MAIN CONSTITUENTS

Acid: geranic; alcohols: geraniol, citrolellol, linalol, myrtenol, terpineol; aldehyde: citral; ketone: methone; phenol: eugenol; terpene: sabinene.

QUALITIES

A relaxing, warming and refreshing scent. Balancing in nature because it stimulates the adrenal cortex, where hormones are produced which regulate the production of hormones in other organs. Geranium has antiseptic, anti-depressant, anti-inflammatory as well as diuretic properties.

TRADITIONAL USES

Geranium is popular as an insect repellent and is used in the cosmetics industry. A very valuable oil for skin care as it can be used on all skin types due to its ability to balance the production of sebum, as well as having an anti-bacterial effect. Geranium is also effective in helping the body to eliminate fluids because of its stimulating effect on the lymphatic system and its diuretic action.

It has been used as an aid for menopausal problems because of its apparent balancing effect on the hormones. Also effective for premenstrual tension as it helps to relieve excessive fluid retention.

CAUTIONS

Generally a non-sensitizing oil, but it may cause irritation to very sensitive skin.

LAVENDER *Lavandula officinalis*;
Lavandula angustifolia; *Lavandula vera*
Middle note; distilled from the flowers

ORIGINS

Native to the Mediterranean region, it is widely distributed in southern Europe. Cultivated primarily in France, Italy and England. *Lavandula* is derived from the Latin 'lavare' which means 'to wash' as it was widely used for bathing. It is also known as *Lavandula angustifolia* and *Lavandula vera* which means 'true lavender'. It is the most versatile of all the essential oils. Used in folk medicine as a mild sedative, cough suppressant, for gastric disturbances and for rheumatic pain. Lavender was used for flavouring food for the purpose of 'comforting the stomach'. A compound tincture of Lavender known as Lavender drops, has been recognized in the *British Herbal Pharmacopoeia* for over 200 years. Lavender oil was used to stimulate paralysed limbs by rubbing it on the affected area. It was used during the Second World War as an antiseptic for swabbing wounds. In France it is not uncommon for a bottle of Lavender essence to be found in the home where it is used as a domestic remedy against bruises, bites and minor aches and pains. Lavender's healing properties when applied to burns were instrumental in introducing the art of aromatherapy to our Western culture.

MAIN CONSTITUENTS

Alcohols: borneol, geraniol, lavandulol, linalol; esters: geranyl acetate, lavandulyl acetate, linalyl acetate; ketone: cineole; sesquiterpene: caryophyllene; terpenes: limonene, pinene.

QUALITIES

One of the most useful of all essential oils. Its actions include normalizing, analgesic, antiseptic, antibiotic, anti-depressant, anti-bacterial, decongestant and sedative effects. It is also a balancing oil and can be used to mentally balance or 'centre' oneself.

TRADITIONAL USES

Widely used in perfumery, especially toilet water, because of its popular scent. Inhaled to prevent vertigo and fainting. As an insect repellent. Used in veterinary practices for killing lice and other parasites on animals.

This is the only oil that can safely be applied neat to the skin, especially for burns. It can be used for all types of skin.

A good inhalant for catarrh, sinusitis, bronchitis and colds in general. It also acts as a nerve sedative. Can be used in the bath for relaxation as well as to help relieve aches and pains. For migraines and headaches 1 drop can be applied directly onto the temples, or it can be used in a cold compress alone, or with 1 drop of Peppermint oil added. Helps prevent scarring while promoting rapid healing.

ROSEMARY *Rosmarinus officinalis*
Middle note; distilled from flowering tops and leaves

ORIGINS

The name means 'dew of the sea' from the Latin 'ros maris'. Native of the Mediterranean region, especially on rocky areas near the sea, it is cultivated throughout the world. Used as an incense for certain religious ceremonies. Mrs Grieve says, in *A Modern Herbal*, that 'A Rosemary branch, richly gilded and tied with silken ribands of all colours, was also presented to wedding guests, as a symbol of love and loyalty'. It was also used at funerals, the custom being to cast a sprig of Rosemary onto the coffin. In Spain and Italy it was considered as a protection against evil spirits. Rosemary, along with Juniper, was burned to purify the air and prevent infection in French hospitals.

MAIN CONSTITUENTS

Alcohols: borneol, linalol; aldehyde: cuminic; ester: bornyl acetate; ketones: camphor, cineole; sesquiterpene: caryophyllene; terpenes: camphene, pinene.

QUALITIES

A strengthening, invigorating oil, which is useful for people who have low blood pressure (are hypotensive).

TRADITIONAL USES

Used for stimulating weak memory, hence the saying from Shakespeare's Hamlet 'There's Rosemary, that's for remembrance'. Also used widely in cooking and as an ingredient in perfumes and other cosmetics, especially shampoo. It is an original ingredient of eau-de-Cologne.

CAUTIONS

Should not be used for people who suffer from high blood pressure or epilepsy because of its stimulating qualities. Avoid use during pregnancy. Not to be used when taking homoeopathic remedies.

TEA TREE *Melaleuca alternifolia*
Top note; distilled from leaves and small branches

ORIGINS

Found only in Australia, Tea Tree is from the same botanical family as Cajeput, Clove Bud, Eucalyptus and Niaouli. As there are many varieties of *Melaleuca*, it is important to ensure that the Tea Tree used in aromatherapy is in fact *alternifolia*. One of the reasons is that the amount of cineole present is not generally high enough to cause skin irritation. A three-year study conducted in Australia by Arthur Penfold, a scientist working for the government in New South Wales, concluded in 1925 that *Melaleuca alternifolia* had antiseptic properties many times stronger than carbolic acid which was the main anti-bacterial agent in use at that time. In addition, it was shown to be non-toxic and non-irritating. Its germicidal potency, with the added attraction of not destroying tissue along with the bacteria, was noted in the early 1930s. It was also noted that Tea Tree acted as a deodorant, immediately clearing away any foul smell from wounds or abscesses.

Tea Tree was so highly regarded that cutters and producers were exempt from service in the Second World War. The Australian government wanted to issue Tea Tree as part of the first-aid kits given to their army and navy. It was impossible, however, for the producers to keep up with the demand and so scientific researchers developed synthetic alternatives. These were not as effective, but, because they were more readily available they eventually replaced the natural product. Consciousness about natural versus synthetic products started to come full circle during the 1960s, and so a renewed interest in Tea Tree emerged and has continued to flourish since.

Tea Tree contains at least forty-eight organic compounds, some of which have rarely, if ever, been found elsewhere in nature. These substances are not particularly effective on their own. But by using the whole plant the maximum healing potential of Tea Tree is reached.

Much study is still under way in Australia which is focusing on a number of potential applications for Tea Tree. One large corporation in Australia periodically uses a controlled dose of the oil by misting it through an air conditioning system. This inhibits mould, fungi and bacteria which usually thrive in warm, moist, dark places such as air ducts. The result is better, cleaner air, less mould on walls and less contamination in general.

This oil has been used for thousands of years by the aboriginal people of Australia. They use the leaves to treat cuts and wounds.

Tea Tree is sometimes incorrectly spelled 'Ti Tree' and this can be confusing as 'Ti' is the Maori name for another tree (sp. Cordyline), which is completely unrelated. When Captain Cook first arrived in Australia the leaves from one of the many species of this plant were used as a substitute tea, hence the name.

MAIN CONSTITUENTS

Alcohol: terpineol; ketone: cineole; terpenes: cymene, pinene, terpinene. Also contains certain constituents which are rarely found in nature such as viridiflorene.

QUALITIES

Has a cooling action; it is the best anti-viral essential oil. It is effective against bacteria and fungi as well as viruses. A very powerful stimulant to the immune system.

TRADITIONAL USES

Has been used by the Bundjalund Aborigines for its incredible healing properties. Its long list of uses include burns, stings, skin irritations (although it can be irritating to some sensitive skin types), vaginal infections, arthritic pain, muscular aches, spasms, gum infections, mouth ulcers, catarrh, cold sores, sore throats and other respiratory complaints.

CAUTIONS

Potentially a skin irritant to some individuals if taken in large dosages.

USING YOUR ESSENTIAL OILS FOR COMMON AILMENTS

Listed below are various 'recipes' for alleviating common ailments at home, using the essential oils provided in this kit. Please refer to chapter three for instructions on how to prepare each treatment before using it.

As a rule essential oils should not be applied to the skin undiluted as they can be irritants. So, you will need to blend most oils with a good quality carrier oil (see pages 65–7) for this use; Lavender is an exception, as we have already seen.

All the definitions for the conditions listed on the following pages are for information purposes only and in no way should be used for self-diagnosis. The use of the essential oils suggested for the conditions mentioned comes from years of research and first-hand experience of a number of people dedicated to using natural products to assist in the healing process. The applications given are to be understood as ways to help alleviate the condition; they are not intended to take the place of medical attention.

ABSCESS

OILS

Lavender, Tea Tree (*choose one or a combination of both*).

APPLICATIONS

In a hot compress placed directly over the swelling.

ACNE

OILS

Geranium, Lavender, Rosemary, Tea Tree (*use one or a blend of two or three, unless otherwise indicated*).

APPLICATIONS

In the bath (*4–6 drops*).

Massage blend, cream or toner applied to the affected area.

Massage blend for the whole body using Rosemary and Geranium which will help stimulate the lymphatic system to clear toxins from the body.

ALOPECIA (Hair Loss)

OILS

Lavender, Rosemary (*choose one or a blend of both*).

APPLICATIONS

In a massage blend applied to the scalp. The scalp should be massaged regularly to help increase blood circulation. This can be done once or twice a week, leaving the oil blend on the hair for at least an hour (and longer if possible) before shampooing it out (a non-alkaline shampoo is recommended for use). Jojoba would be a good choice of carrier oil for the massage blend as it is the least greasy of the carrier oils as well as being nourishing for the scalp and hair.

Note: Although the above treatment can be effective for temporary hair loss due to injury or disease, hereditary baldness may not respond in the same way.

APHTHA (MOUTH ULCERS)

OILS

Geranium

APPLICATIONS

In a gargle (*1 drop in $\frac{1}{3}$ of a glass of warm water*).

ARTHRITIS

OILS

Lavender, Rosemary, Tea Tree

APPLICATIONS

In the bath (*4–6 drops*).

Use a blend to massage the affected area.

Apply a warm compress to the affected area.

ATHLETE'S FOOT

OILS

Lavender, Tea Tree (*use a single oil or a blend*).

APPLICATIONS

In the bath (*4–6 drops*).

In a cream.

BABY'S COMPLAINTS

OILS

Lavender

APPLICATIONS

Dilute 1 drop of Lavender in either almond oil or whole milk. Disperse the blend into the

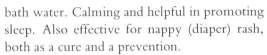

bath water. Calming and helpful in promoting sleep. Also effective for nappy (diaper) rash, both as a cure and a prevention.

For coughs and colds, a single drop of Lavender can be placed on the sheet in baby's cot or a few drops added to water in a burner alongside, but not within reach of, the cot.

For restlessness try adding a single drop of Lavender to night clothes.

A drop of Lavender can also be effective for teething and, when diluted with almond oil, can be gently massaged onto babies' cheeks.

BLISTERS

OILS

Lavender

APPLICATIONS

Several drops of Lavender can be placed on a piece of gauze which is then placed over the blister. Large blisters can be punctured first with a sterilized needle. Be sure that the gauze is not so thick that it prevents air from reaching the blister.

BOILS

OILS

Lavender, Tea Tree (*use a single oil or blend of the two*).

APPLICATIONS

The area around the boil should be cleansed several times a day. Several drops of essential oil or essential oil blend can be added to a sink of warm water for this purpose. Make sure that the water is well agitated to disperse the essential oil.

In the bath (*4–6 drops*).

BRONCHITIS (ACUTE)

OILS

Eucalyptus, Lavender, Rosemary (*choose one or use a blend of two or all three*).

APPLICATIONS

In a hot compress applied to the chest area.

In a massage blend applied to the chest area.

BURNS

OILS

Lavender

APPLICATIONS

Apply neat Lavender essential oil directly onto a minor burn. It will reduce the pain as well as promote healing. For a large burn, Lavender can be poured onto a sterile gauze which is then applied to the burnt area. The gauze can be changed periodically. Of course, severe burns will require qualified medical assistance.

BURSITIS

OILS

Lavender

APPLICATIONS

In the bath (*4–6 drops*).

In a hot compress applied directly over the problem area.

In a massage blend applied gently over the problem area.

CATARRH

OILS

Eucalyptus, Lavender, Tea Tree (*choose one or a*

blend of two or all three).

APPLICATIONS

In the bath (*4–6 drops*).
Place a few drops on a tissue and inhale as required.
In a fragrancer.
In a massage blend applied to the chest area.

CHILBLAINS

OILS

Rosemary

APPLICATIONS
(TO HELP IMPROVE CIRCULATION)

In the bath (*4–6 drops*).
Massage blend using 1 drop for each 5 ml of carrier oil. Apply sparingly to affected area.

COLDS AND FLU

OILS

Eucalyptus, Lavender, Tea Tree (*use one or a blend of two or all three).*

APPLICATIONS

In a bath (*4–6 drops*) at the first sign of cold or flu.
In a steam inhalation.
In a fragrancer.

COUGHS

OILS

Eucalyptus, Lavender (*choose one).*

APPLICATIONS

In a steam inhalation.
In a massage blend and gently massaged on the throat and chest area.
In a fragrancer.

CUTS

OILS

Eucalyptus, Lavender, Tea Tree (*choose one).*

APPLICATIONS

A cool compress can be applied to the cut area.
Apply a cream directly to the cut.

CYSTITIS

OILS

Eucalyptus, Lavender, Tea Tree (*choose one or use a blend of two or all three).*

APPLICATIONS

In the bath (*4–6 drops*).
In a massage blend applied gently over the abdomenal area.

DANDRUFF

OILS

Rosemary, Tea Tree (*use a single oil).*

APPLICATIONS

One or 2 drops can be added directly to a capful of shampoo. Two drops of Rosemary essential oil and 2 tablespoons of apple cider vinegar (organic if possible) can be added to 1 litre lukewarm water. This can be used as a final rinse after shampooing. Be sure to disperse the essential oil before application.

DEHYDRATED SKIN

OILS

Geranium, Lavender (*use a single oil or blend of the two).*

APPLICATIONS

In a facial, cream or massage blend. Apply gently to the skin surface.

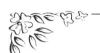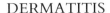
DERMATITIS

OILS

Geranium, Lavender, Tea Tree (*choose one oil or a blend of two or all three*).

APPLICATIONS

A cold compress is especially effective if the skin is itchy.

In the bath (*4–6 drops*).

In a cream applied directly to the skin.

DISINFECTANT

OILS

Tea Tree

APPLICATIONS

Add several drops to warm water for washing floors and other surfaces.

EARACHE

OILS

Lavender

APPLICATIONS

A hot compress with Lavender oil can be used to help alleviate the pain; however, proper medical attention should be sought to determine the precise cause, particularly if the problem persists or if there are other associated symptoms.

ECZEMA

OILS

Geranium, Lavender, Tea Tree (*choose one oil or a blend of two or all three*).

APPLICATIONS

A cold compress, especially for itchy skin.

In the bath (*4–6 drops*).

In a cream applied directly to the skin.

FEVERS

OILS

Eucalyptus, Lavender, Rosemary, Tea Tree (*choose one or use up to three oils in a blend*).

APPLICATIONS

In a bath (*4–6 drops*).

In a cold compress applied to the forehead.

In a fragrancer.

In a massage blend applied to the chest area.

HAIR CARE

OILS

Lavender

APPLICATIONS

Place several drops in the palm of your hand, rub your hands together and run your hands through your hair starting at the scalp. This can be done to dry hair before brushing or combing in the morning or applied just before going to bed at night. This helps to sort out knots and tangles while leaving the hair beautifully fragranced.

HAY FEVER

OILS

Eucalyptus, Lavender (*choose one oil or a blend of both*).

APPLICATIONS

In a steam inhalation.

A few drops on a tissue inhaled as required.

In a massage blend used in general massage.

HEADACHE

OILS

Eucalyptus, Lavender, Rosemary (*choose*

Lavender alone or in combination with Rosemary for general purposes. Eucalyptus can be effective if the headache is connected with catarrh or a sinus infection).

APPLICATIONS

A cold compress over the forehead and temples can be very effective.

A drop of Lavender can be rubbed undiluted on each temple.

Use in a fragrancer.

Put several drops on a tissue and inhale with deep breaths, as required.

INSECT BITES

OILS

Geranium, Lavender, Tea Tree *(choose one oil or a blend of two or all three unless otherwise indicated).*

APPLICATIONS

One drop of Lavender can be applied neat to the affected area.

In the bath *(4–6 drops).*

As a local wash to the affected area.

INSECT REPELLENT

OILS

Eucalyptus, Geranium, Lavender, Tea Tree *(choose one oil or a blend of two or three).*

APPLICATIONS

As a spray *(use 4 drops of essential oil or essential oil blend to $\frac{1}{2}$ litre (1 pt) warm water).* Spray around windows, doors, garden furniture, campsite or any place you may want to deter insects.

For the body, use a blend using 10 ml carrier oil to 4 drops of essential oil, or a combination of essential oils, applied directly to the exposed parts of your skin.

INSOMNIA

OILS

Lavender

APPLICATIONS

In the bath *(4–6 drops).*

In a fragrancer.

Place a few drops on the pillow or night clothes.

Use in a massage blend applied to the abdomen, chest and forehead.

MIGRAINE

OILS

Lavender

APPLICATIONS

A cold compress can be very helpful, especially at the early or pre-migraine stage.

MORNING SICKNESS

OILS

Lavender

APPLICATIONS

A few drops on a tissue inhaled as required.

MUSCULAR ACHES AND PAINS

OILS

Eucalyptus, Lavender, Rosemary, Tea Tree *(choose one oil or a blend of two or three).*

APPLICATIONS

In the bath *(4–6 drops).*

In a massage blend applied to problem area.

NASAL CONGESTION

OILS

Eucalyptus

APPLICATIONS

In a steam inhalation.
Place several drops on a tissue and inhale.
Several drops can be sprinkled on the pillow.
In a fragrancer.

PRE-MENSTRUAL TENSION

OILS

Geranium, Rosemary (*choose Geranium unless otherwise indicated*).

APPLICATIONS

In the bath (*4–6 drops*).
In a hot compress applied to the abdomen.
In a massage blend a mixture of Geranium and Rosemary can help fluid retention.

RHEUMATISM

OILS

Eucalyptus, Rosemary, Tea Tree (*choose one oil or a blend of two or all three*).

APPLICATIONS

In the bath (*4–6 drops*).
In a hot compress applied directly on to the affected area.
In a massage blend applied to the affected area.

SEBORRHOEA

OILS

Geranium, Lavender, Tea Tree (*choose one oil or a blend of two or all three*).

APPLICATIONS

In the bath (*4–6 drops*).

In a cream applied directly to the affected area.

SORE THROAT

OILS

Lavender

APPLICATIONS

One drop with warm water for gargling.
In a steam inhalation.
In a massage applied to the throat area.

STRETCH MARKS

OILS

Lavender

APPLICATIONS

In a massage blend gently apply to the affected area. This can be done daily.

SWELLING

OILS

Geranium, Tea Tree

APPLICATIONS

In a massage blend stroking the affected area in the direction of the heart.

THRUSH

OILS

Lavender, Tea Tree (*choose Lavender or use a blend of both with Lavender being dominant*).

APPLICATIONS

In the bath (*4–6 drops*).
As a local wash.

TIRED FEET

OILS

Lavender

APPLICATIONS

In a foot-bath.

VAGINAL INFECTION
OILS
Lavender, Tea Tree (*use Lavender alone or use a blend of both with Lavender being dominant*).
APPLICATIONS
In the bath (*4–6 drops*).
As a local wash.

VARICOSE VEINS
OILS
Lavender

APPLICATIONS

In the bath (*4–6 drops*).
In a cream applied directly above (not over) the varicose vein(s).

WOUNDS
OILS
Lavender, Tea Tree
APPLICATIONS
A few drops of either Lavender or Tea Tree placed on a plaster which is applied to the affected area.
In a cold compress applied directly on the affected area.

OTHER USES OF OILS IN THIS KIT

Fragrance has a powerful effect on the mind. Just walking through an English garden in full bloom can have a dramatic effect on emotions. The profusion of colour plays a part but the smells send direct messages to the brain. This is why it is important that you really like the smell of an essential oil if it is to have a positive effect. Listed below are some suggestions, based on the essential oils provided in your *Aromatherapy Kit*, which can enhance the atmosphere and mood as appropriate.

BALANCING
OILS
Geranium, Lavender (*choose one oil or a blend of both*).
APPLICATIONS
In the bath (*4–6 drops*).

In a fragrancer.
In a massage blend for overall body massage or specific areas such as the neck and shoulders. Try massaging some of the blend into the soles of the feet as well.
Place several drops on a tissue and inhale as required.
In a perfume.

CALMING AND SEDATIVE
OILS
Lavender
APPLICATIONS
In a bath (*4–6 drops*).
In a fragrancer.
In a massage blend for overall body massage or for specific areas such as the neck and shoulders. Try massaging some of the blend

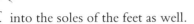

into the soles of the feet as well.

As a perfume: a few drops can be placed on a tissue or piece of cotton wool and tucked inside clothing.

CLARITY AND MEMORY ENHANCER

OILS

Rosemary

APPLICATIONS

In a fragrancer.

Apply several drops to a tissue and inhale.

INVIGORATING

OILS

Eucalyptus, Rosemary

APPLICATIONS

In the bath (*4–6 drops*).

In a fragrancer.

In a massage blend for overall body massage or for specific areas such as the neck and shoulders; can be massaged into the soles of the feet as well.

TENSION RELIEF

OILS

Geranium, Lavender (*choose one or use a blend of the two*).

APPLICATIONS

In the bath (*4–6 drops*).

In a fragrancer.

Place several drops on a tissue and inhale.

In a massage blend for overall body massage or for specific areas such as the neck and shoulders; can also be massaged into the soles of the feet.

IN CONCLUSION

You have now been introduced to a variety of applications for the oils in your kit. And diligent study of the information in this book should suggest more varied uses to you. As you become more experienced, you will want to increase your range of oils and thus the range of applications in order to tailor your aromatherapy treatments to your personal needs. Please ensure that you only use aromatherapy-quality essential oils. Oils with the Aromark seal have that guarantee (see 'Useful Addresses', page 111).

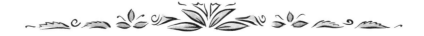

GLOSSARY

Acne A skin disorder in which the sebaceous glands become inflamed. Results in pimples, blackheads and whiteheads and, in severe cases, pus-filled cysts under the skin.

Alopecia An absence of hair from areas where it normally grows. This may be due to disease or injury.

Antigen Any substance that the body regards as foreign or potentially dangerous.

Aphtha A small ulcer thought to be caused by infection. Usually occurs in the mouth in groups of white or red spots.

Arthritis Inflammation of one or more joints, characterized by swelling, a burning sensation, redness of the overlying skin, pain and restriction of motion. Usually caused by a build up of uric acid, which gets deposited, in crystalline form, in the joints.

Asthma Condition characterized by sudden spasms of the bronchi, which make breathing difficult.

Boil A tender, inflamed area of skin containing pus. Usually caused by bacteria entering through a hair follicle or a break in the skin.

Bronchitis Inflammation of the bronchi (air passages beyond the windpipe),

usually caused by virus or bacteria.

Bronchospasm A narrowing of bronchi by muscular contraction, which occurs in response to certain stimuli.

Bursitis Inflammation of a bursa (small sac of fibrous tissue around joints), which can result from injury or infection. Usually painful, and can restrict movement of a nearby joint.

Carminative A substance that relieves flatulence.

Chilblains A red, round, itchy swelling of the skin occurring in cold weather, generally on the fingers or toes.

Cystitis Inflammation of the urinary bladder usually caused by infection.

Dermatitis Inflammation of the skin in which it can become red and itchy and small blisters may develop.

Eczema A superficial inflammation of the skin mainly affecting the epidermis.

Epidermis The outer layer of the skin, itself divided into four layers.

Hypotensive Having abnormally low blood pressure.

Intestinal tract The part of the alimentary canal that extends from the stomach to the anus.

Keratinization Process by which cells become horny due to the deposition of keratin (a fibrous protein).

Migraine A recurrent, throbbing headache that tends to affect one side of the head. Sometimes there is a forewarning consisting of flickering, bright lights or blurring of vision, which clears as the headache develops.

Officinalis Officially used for medicinal purposes.

Palpitation An awareness of the heartbeat. In normal circumstances, this can be the result of fear, exertion or strong emotion.

Psoriasis A chronic skin disease, caused by keratinization of the skin cells. Scaly, red patches form on the elbows, forearms, knees, legs, scalp and other parts of the body causing irritation.

Rheumatism Any disorder in which aching affects the muscles and joints.

Sebaceous gland Any simple or branched gland in the skin that secretes an oily substance known as sebum.

Seborrhoea An excessive secretion of sebum by the sebaceous glands. The glands are enlarged, especially beside the nose and other parts of the face.

Spasm A sustained, involuntary muscular contraction.

Stimulant An agent that promotes the activity of a body system or function.

Unguent A soothing or healing salve.

BIBLIOGRAPHY

Berkson, Devaki. *The Foot Book*, Savage M D, Barnes & Noble Books, 1977

Culpeper, Nicholas. *Culpeper's Complete Herbal & English Physician*, J Gleave and Son, 1826 (reproduction 1981)

Davis, Patricia. *Aromatherapy: An A–Z*, Saffron Walden, C W Daniel, 1988

Devereux, Charla. *Nutrition and Diet Logic*, Slough, Foulsham, 1992

El Mahdy, Christine. *Mummies: Myth and Magic*, London, Thames & Hudson, 1989

Fabricius, Johannes. *Alchemy*, London, Aquarian Press, 1989

Genders, Roy. *Natural Beauty*, Exeter, Webb & Bower, 1985

Grieve, Mrs M. *A Modern Herbal*, Vols. I & II, New York, Dover Books, 1971

Heinerman, John. *Science of Herbal*

Medicine, Utah, Bi-World, 1979

Hoffmann, David. *The Holistic Herbal*, Shaftesbury, Element Books, 1988

Lad, Vasant Dr. *Ayurveda*, 2nd edn, Detroit MI, Lotus Press, 1985

Lawless, Julia. *The Encyclopaedia of Essential Oils*, Shaftesbury, Element Books, 1992

Leung, Albert Y. *Chinese Herbal Remedies*, New York, Universe Books, 1984

Lidell, Lucinda. *The Book of Massage*, London, Ebury Press, 1984

Martin, Gill. *Aromatherapy*, London, Optima, 1989

Mulherin, Jennifer. *Spices and Natural Flavourings*, London, Ward Lock, 1988

Natural Oils Research Association. *The Art of Smelling Essential Oils*, Windsor,

Natural Oils Research Association

Price, Shirley. *Practical Aromatherapy*, Wellingborough, Thorsons, 1987

Puharich, Andrija. *Beyond Telepathy*, London, Picador, 1975

Schnaubelt, Kurt. 'Friendly molecules', Vol. II, no. 2, p.20 and Vol. II, no. 3, in *The International Journal of Aromatherapy*, Summer & Autumn, Hove, 1989

Sellar, Wanda. *The Directory of Essential Oils*, Saffron Walden, C W Daniel, 1992

Shaukat, Sidra. *Skin and Body Care*, Shaftesbury, Element, 1992

Stuart, Malcolm (Ed.). *Herbs and Herbalism*, New York, Crescent Books, 1979

Thorwald, Jurgen. *Science and Secrets of*

Early Medicine, London, Thames & Hudson, 1962

Tisserand, Maggie. *Aromatherapy for Women*, Wellingborough, Thorsons, 1985

Tisserand, Robert. *The Art of Aromatherapy*, Saffron Walden,

C W Daniel, 1988

Ullman, Dana. *Homoeopathy, Medicine for the 21st Century*, Wellingborough, Thorsons, 1988

Unterman, Alan. *Dictionary of Jewish Lore & Legend*, London, Thames & Hudson, 1991

Valnet, Dr Jean. *The Practice of Aromatherapy*, Saffron Walden, C W Daniel, 1988

Watt, Martin. *Plant Aromatics: A Data & Reference Manual*, Witham, Martin Watt

Yeoh, Aileen. *Longevity*, Singapore, Times Books, 1989

USEFUL ADDRESSES

When requesting information from any of these organizations, a stamped, self-addressed envelope is always appreciated.

UNITED KINGDOM

Aromatherapy Organisations Council, 3 Latymer Close, Braybrooke, Market Harborough, Leics. LE16 8LN
The Council, which incorporates almost all of the aromatherapy groups in UK, has recently been set up to oversee standards.
Empress, P O Box 92, Penzance, Cornwall TR18 2BX
For essential oils and carrier oils. All essential oils sold by Empress have the Aromark seal. Also contact Charla Devereux, Transatlantic Co-ordinator for the Natural Oils Research Association (NORA) for information about NORA and research into essential oils.
Essential Oils Trade Association, 61 Clinton Lane, Kenilworth, Warwicks. CV8 1AS
For essential oils and carrier oils.

International Federation of Aromatherapists (IFA), Department of Continuing Education, Royal Masonic Hospital, Ravenscourt Park, London W6 0TN
Send a SAE for a list of accredited training schools or IFA members in your area.
Natural Oils Research Association, P O Box No 1604, Windsor, Berks. SL4 3YR
Runs educational courses (Birkbeck College, London) and carries out analysis and testing (Aromark) of essential oils. Also publishes technical and general papers.

UNITED STATES

Charla Devereux, Transatlantic Co-ordinator, Natural Oils Research Association (NORA), P O Box 92, Penzance, Cornwall TR18 2BX, United Kingdom
For information about aromatherapy and the US organisation for overseeing standards of essential oils (being set up at the time of going to press).

Ms. Dina Khader, 491 Lexington Avenue, Mount Kisco, New York 10549
For essential oils carrying the Aromark seal and for information on aromatherpy and essential oils.
Rev. Claire L. North, North Lights, 329 West 89th Street, Apartment 2, New York City, New York 10024
For essential oils carrying the Aromark seal.

AUSTRALIA

W. Cowan, 4/25 Billyard Avenue, Elizabeth Bay, NSW 2011, Australia
For information on aromatherapy and essential oils.

ACKNOWLEDGEMENTS

Although I have been fascinated by plants since childhood, I really must thank John Steele for sparking off my interest in essential oils. My work with them began in 1988 as the result of a chance meeting with Lorna Rappaport and John Potter. It was the assistance and support of John and Barbara Dower, and Margaret James, however, that enabled me to establish my own company. There have been numerous other people along the way who have encouraged, supported and contributed to my knowledge and understanding of aromatherapy, both directly and through their books. Special thanks to Lieve Reynolds, an aromatherapist with a truly gentle touch. Hugh Deynem and Sue Bartlett's assistance with the massage section is also greatly appreciated. And thanks go to Ian Jackson, whose enthusiasm allowed this work to happen in the first place, and Zoë Hughes for her editorial support and overall encouragement. I appreciate the help of my husband, Paul, in reading through the manuscript. But it is to Bernie Hephrun, consultant for this book, that I owe my greatest thanks. His wealth of knowledge and readiness to share it has been a most valued contribution.

EDDISON · SADD EDITIONS

Editor Zoë Hughes
Art Director Elaine Partington
Designer Pritilata Ramjee
Illustrator Julie Carpenter
Proofreaders Marilyn Inglis and Kirsty Wheeler
Indexer Peter Moloney
Production Charles James and Hazel Kirkman

INDEX

abscess 102
acids 18
acne 22, 71, 102
alcohols 18
aldehydes 18
allergies 79
alopecia 102
anxiety 92–3
aphtha (mouth ulcers) 102
Aromark seal 25
aromatherapists, qualified 49–50
aromatherapy, history of 9
arthritis 102
asthma 79
athlete's foot 102

Basil 21, 27, 93
bathing treatments 61–3
beauty treatments 57–60, 68–72, 75–6
  oil application charts 73–5
Benzoin Resinoid 27
Bergamot 28, 47
Black Pepper 21, 28–9
blister 103
blood pressure 83
boils 103
bronchitis 80, 82, 103
burns 103
bursitis 103

Cajeput 29, 61
Camphor 29–30
Caraway 30
carrier oils 20, 47, 57, 65–7, 70, 78
catarrh 103–4
Cedarwood 10–11, 30
cellulite 81–2
Chamomile 16, 19, 22, 31, 80, 83
chilblains 70, 104
children and babies 47–8, 81, 102–3
Cinnamon Leaf 31–2
Clary Sage 18, 22, 32, 76, 82, 93
Clove Bud 32, 93
colds 104
compresses 60–1, 80, 82
Coriander 10, 33
coughs 104
creams, face 57–8

cuts 104
Cypress 33
cystitis 104

dandruff 76, 104
depression 92
dermatitis 105
diarrhoea 81

earache 79, 105
eczema 70, 105
essential oils 16–17, 27–44
  analgesic 78–9
  and emotions 92–3, 108–9
  anti-allergenic 79
  anti-inflammatory 79–80
  antiseptic 80
  anti-spasmodic 80–1
  aperitifs 81
  astringent 81
  blending 51, 59–60, 66–7, 72, 78
  carminative 81
  caution in use of 21–2
  chemical properties 18–19
  deodorant 70
  detoxifying 81–2
  disinfectant 105
  diuretics 82
  emmenagogues 22, 47, 82
  expectorants 82
  extraction methods 11, 12, 19–21
  febrifuge 82–3
  fungicidal 83
  galactagogues 83
  healing properties 22–3
  hypertensive 83
  hypotensive 83
  nervines 83
  purity of 24–5
  skin irritants 46
  storage and care of 48
  synthetic 24
  tonics 83
esters 18
Eucalyptus 97–8

facial treatments 54–5, 57–9, 70, 71, 72
Fennel 23, 33–4, 83
fevers 82–3, 105
flu 104
foot treatments 56, 61–3,

107–8
Frankincense 8, 10, 34, 93

gargles 61
Geranium 16, 18, 82, 98
Ginger 18, 34–5, 93

hair care 59, 75–6, 105
hay fever 105
headache 79, 105–6
health treatments 60–1, 77–83, 91–3
  oil application charts 84–90, 94–5
homoeopathy 14, 21, 22
hormones 23, 92, 98
Hyssop 18, 35

inflammation 79–80
inhalation treatment 61
insect bites 106
insect repellents 64, 106
insomnia 93, 106

Jasmine 35
Juniper Berry 10, 21, 22, 24–5, 35–6

ketones 18

Lavender 12, 13, 16, 18, 21, 22, 52, 69, 78, 98–9, 101, 103
Lemon 18, 23, 36
Lemongrass 18, 36–7

Mandarin 37
Marjoram 22, 37
massage 13, 14, 49–50, 51–6, 78, 81, 83
Melissa 18, 37–8, 70
menopause 23
menstruation 22, 47, 82, 98, 107
migraine 79, 106
milk, breast 83
morning sickness 80, 106
muscular pain 106
Myrrh 10, 17, 38

nasal congestion 107
Neroli 18, 21, 38–9
Niaouli 39
Nutmeg 39–40

Orange 40, 62

Patchouli 8, 17, 40, 48
Peppermint 13, 16, 18, 40–1, 61, 63, 93
perfumes 25, 59–60
Petitgrain 41
phenols 18–19
Pine Needle 41
pregnancy 47, 82
psoriasis 71

reflexology 62–3
rheumatism 107
room fragrancers 63–4
Rose Absolute 41–2
Rose Otto 17, 41–2, 48
Rosemary 12, 18, 76, 83, 93, 99–100
rosewater 12, 21
Rosewood 18, 42

Sage 18, 42–3
Sandalwood 17, 43
seborrhoea 71, 107
sebum 16, 69, 71
sesquiterpenes 19
skin care 69–75, 104
  oil application charts 73–5
  skin sensitivity 46–7, 71–2
  skin types 70–2
smell, sense of 7–9, 13
spasms 80–1
steam treatments 60, 61, 80
stress 71, 72, 78, 81, 92–3
stretch marks 107
swelling 107

Tagetes 43
Tarragon 43–4
Tea Tree 18, 100–1
terpenes 19
throat, sore 79, 107
thrush 83, 107
Thyme 16, 19, 44, 83
toners 59
travel sickness 80

vaginal infection 108
varicose veins 81, 108

wounds 108

Ylang Ylang 16, 17, 44